Wine, Chocolate, & Your Good Health

Joe Urbach
www.gardeningaustin.com
www.phytonutrientfarms.com

A

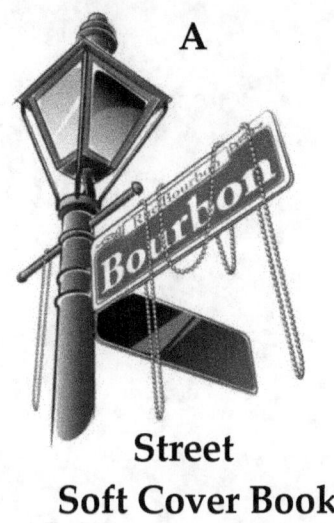

Street
Soft Cover Book

1st published in the United State in 2017 by
Bond Street Publications, a Hojo Enterprises Company

1st Printing 2017

Copyright © Joseph Urbach 2017

DEDICATION

This book was written for my
wife Holly and for all of us who
love to sit back and enjoy a little
bit of life's finest pleasures -
chocolate and wine!

Just to give us another reason to
indulge!

CONTENTS

Forward

I am not a scientist, nor a medical doctor, nor a nutritionist nor any other kind of healthcare worker. I am not a research professional nor have I ever been involved in medical research of any kind.

I am a gardener, a father, a grandfather, and a diabetic. All of this led me to my concern about nutrition, and in turn, led me on a quest that eventually led to the writing of this my **_Yes, Food IS Medicine_** series of books. My journey of exploration has convinced me that there is a very serious problem with the fruit and vegetables that are finding their way into our local markets and eventually on to our dinner plates. The real concern is that it soon can impact our health. In addition, half of the children on planet Earth live in poverty conditions, many suffering malnutrition and forced to drink polluted or tainted water. In this day and age, with all the modern advances of man, this situation is completely unacceptable and that is why I had to write that series.

So, like many of you, I set off in search of helpful health information – but alas, most of what I found was of little merit and even less use. I found misinformation, false information and outright lies. Much of the worst of the 'garbage' info I found concerned chocolate, beer, and wine – three of my favorite things - and so this book was just begging to be written! The information I present in this work is provided for your consideration only and I absolutely do not condone, endorse, or recommend that you take up drinking alcohol or stuffing yourself with candy bars, or even change any of your diet or exercise habits without first consulting your healthcare professional.

My honest belief is that knowledge is power and my goal is to empower you with the information that follows so that you and your doctor can choose the best course of action for you to take to help you achieve a better, healthier, happier, and longer life!

I Am Not A Doctor

The information presented here is accurate to the best of my knowledge.

I am not a doctor therefore this information is not intended to diagnose, treat, cure or prevent any disease because only doctors can do that.

Please do your own research!

Let me say right up front at the beginning of this book that too much of a good thing is not a good thing! Increased alcohol consumption over time will not lead to better health but could, in fact, ruin your health. What's more the same is true for the unchecked consumption of chocolate!

Moderation is the key word here! Keep that in mind as you read on.

INTRODUCTION

I am sure each of you has heard, as I so often do, that eating chocolate, and drinking wine, are basically bad for your mind and body, and from a health standpoint should be avoided.

Well the more research I do into food and drink and how they relate to our health and nutrition the more I discovered the truth. That truth is that the thought of almost any food or drink as inherently bad for us is just plain hogwash!

Chocolate and wine are not at all bad for us, and in fact, offer many health benefits when consumed in moderation! Moderation in our consumption and enjoyment of these, as with so much in life, is the real key.

But how much is considered moderate and how much is too much? How have these two 'notorious baddies' influenced mankind throughout history? Just what health benefits do each of these have to offer us?

Those were the very questions I set out to answer as I sat at my computer one morning to write a post for my Phytonutrient Blog. I started researching and writing and before I knew it I was no longer writing a blog post but had just discovered what my next book was going to be about! The result is in your hands. I hope you enjoy reading it as much as I enjoyed writing it!

Sit back, pour a nice glass of wine, or grab a salted chocolate and enjoy!

1. Chocolate's Early History

"In our modern world, chocolate finds its way onto even the most simplistic dessert menus; there to satisfy the sweetest sweet-tooth. That was not the case in the past. In ancient Mesoamerica, chocolate was deemed a specialty food, achieving a sacred status and reserved for only the wealthiest of people."   - The Phytonutrient Blog

Not too long ago, on a sunny morning in San Francisco's Mission District, half a dozen men and women scooted around a tiny chocolate factory, wrapping bars, checking temperature settings, sorting beans, and prepared to make chocolate candy. Cacao beans that have been fermented, dried, roasted, shelled, and ground tumbled with sugar in a row of shiny metal mixers. After three days of gentle mixing, the buttery smooth results would be transferred to a tempering machine to shape the cacao's natural fat molecules into stable crystal structures. I am talking about the home of a small-batch chocolate maker, Dandelion Chocolate, founded in 2010 by two entrepreneurs and former tech guys. The tools and flavors have changed, but the work of roasting and grinding fermented cacao beans, and mixing them with a few simple ingredients to create a divine food stuff, is a practice that goes back to early Mesoamerican civilizations.

The Olmecs of southern Mexico were probably the first to ferment, roast, and grind cacao beans for drinks and gruels, possibly as early as 1500 BC, said Hayes Lavis, a cultural arts curator for the Smithsonian's National Museum of the American Indian. "There is no written history for the Olmecs," he said, but pots and vessels uncovered from this ancient civilization show traces of the cacao chemical theobromine.

"When you think of chocolate, most people don't think of Mesoamerica. They think of Belgian chocolate," says Lavis. "There's so much rich Central American chocolate history that we're just beginning to understand."

In their raw state, plucked from tangy-sweet, gummy white flesh lining a large pod shaped like a Nerf football, cacao seeds are bitter and unrecognizable as chocolate to a modern American palate. "How would you think to take the seed, harvest it, dry it, let it ferment, and roast it? It's not something you would normally think to do, so how did the ancient peoples of Mesopotamia figure it out?" Lavis pondered. Perhaps, one theory holds, someone was eating the fruit and spitting seeds into the fire, and the rich smell of the roasting beans inspired the thought that "maybe there's something more we could do with this."

The naturally bitter flavor of cacao came through at full strength in early Maya recipes. "This was before they had really good roasting techniques, before they had conching, which is a step that mellows out the flavors, and before they started looking at genetics," says Dandelion co-founder Todd Masonis.

So it seems that some unsung Central American probably deserves the credit for discovering how to ferment and roast cacao beans a millennium or two ago, most likely by accident. Unfortunately, his (or her) name is lost to history but the legacy of their discovery lives on!

In time, chocolate attained a holy status among the ancient inhabitants of Central America and Mexico. "The cacao tree was the embodiment of the Earth's treasures and spiritually represented a link between Earth and the Gods and heavens," wrote entomologist and chocolate expert Allen Young of the Milwaukee Public Museum in "*The Chocolate Tree*"

"Rarely did they add any sweetener — once in a while honey, but mainly the sweetener was only added to try to ferment it," says anthropologist Joel Palka, of the University of Illinois at Chicago. A variety of herbs were on hand, however, for seasoning cacao-based food and drink. "There were literally dozens of things that would be used to flavor it," says Lavis, ranging from chili and vanilla to magnolia.

In traditional preparation methods, which are still used by some small-scale producers, farmers take seeds out of the pods and ferment them in a leaf-covered pile. In more modern methods, the seeds are fermented in raised wooden boxes which enable aeration, drainage, and more consistent results. Dandelion acquires beans that have been fermented for several days and then dried. While the company pours dried beans into a modified coffee roaster carefully calibrated for each type of bean, traditional cacao roasters would have simply placed the beans on a fire or covered them with hot coals. "They'll get almost burnt," Masonis says.

The history of chocolate has a record that goes back nearly 4,000 years. Chocolate was one of the most desired foods of Mesoamerica and was consumed by the Olmec, Maya, and Aztec civilizations, among others. Its consumption even spread, via trade routes, to other parts of the Americas including the Chaco, which reached into modern-day New Mexico.

Cacao figured into pre-modern Maya society as a sacred food, a sign of prestige, a social centerpiece, and a cultural touchstone. "You would have to get together to prepare the chocolate," Palka said. "It's the whole social process." Around Chiapas, Mexico, Palka co-directs an archaeological project focused on Maya culture on the frontier of the Spanish empire. To this day, he encounters people in the area who grow chocolate as a family tradition and cultural practice. "Like coffee in the Arab world, or beer in northern and Eastern Europe, it's not only something that's good, but it is a real part of their identity," he says.

Cacao drinks in Mesoamerica became associated with high status and special occasions, Palka said, like a fine French wine or a craft beer today. Special occasions might include initiation rites for young men or celebrations marking the end of the Maya calendar year.

After the Olmecs, the Maya of Guatemala, Yucatan, and the surrounding region incorporated cacao seed into religious life. Paintings recovered from the time show cacao in mythological scenes and even court proceedings. In the early 12th century, chocolate was used to seal the marriage of the Mixtec ruler '8 Deer' at Monte Albán, a sacred site in the Valley of Oaxaca. "It's one of the few food crops that was used as a dowry or part of wedding ceremonies," Lavis said. Early records of Maya marriages in Guatemala, he added, indicate that in some places, "a woman would have to make the cacao and prove that she could make it with the proper froth before she was allowed to marry."

"When they had to communicate with their gods related to nature, rain, and the fertility of the earth, I'm sure they were pulling cacao out and drinking," Palka said. Many vessels uncovered in the ruins of Maya buildings and burial sites have cacao residues in them, Palka said. "A lot of cacao pots were buried with people," he said, but it is unclear whether people were simply buried with their dishes, or if these pots were involved in funeral ceremonies.

The Maya and the Aztecs believed that cacao was discovered by the gods in a mountain and was then given to the people following their creation. The Maya held a yearly festival to honor the cacao god, Ek Chuah, which included several offerings and rituals to him.

Around Chiapas, Palka said, residents prepared a chocolate drink as an offering for gods related to nature as recently as 1980. "It was something that people enjoyed," he said, "and so they were convinced that their gods enjoyed it, too. And why not?"

Cocoa is thought to have its origin in the Amazon way back in prehistory around about 2000 BC. Today, the tree grows on small farms in West Africa, Southeast Asia, and North and Central America. While different groups were originally trying to use cacao to make beer, chocolate was the result. Lucky for us!

Chocolate is made from the beans of cacao pods from the *Theobroma cacao* tree (actually native to South America) which was first cultivated in extensive orchards near the Pacific and Gulf coasts of central America, especially in the Xoconusco region and the valleys of the Sarstoon, Polochic, and Motagua Rivers (modern Guatemala and Belize), where the tree thrives in the warm and humid climate. There were, in fact, four varieties of cacao bean or *cacahuatl*, as the Aztecs knew them. About six years after planting, the tree produces fruits shaped like small footballs growing directly from the trunk or large branches. Each fruit contains

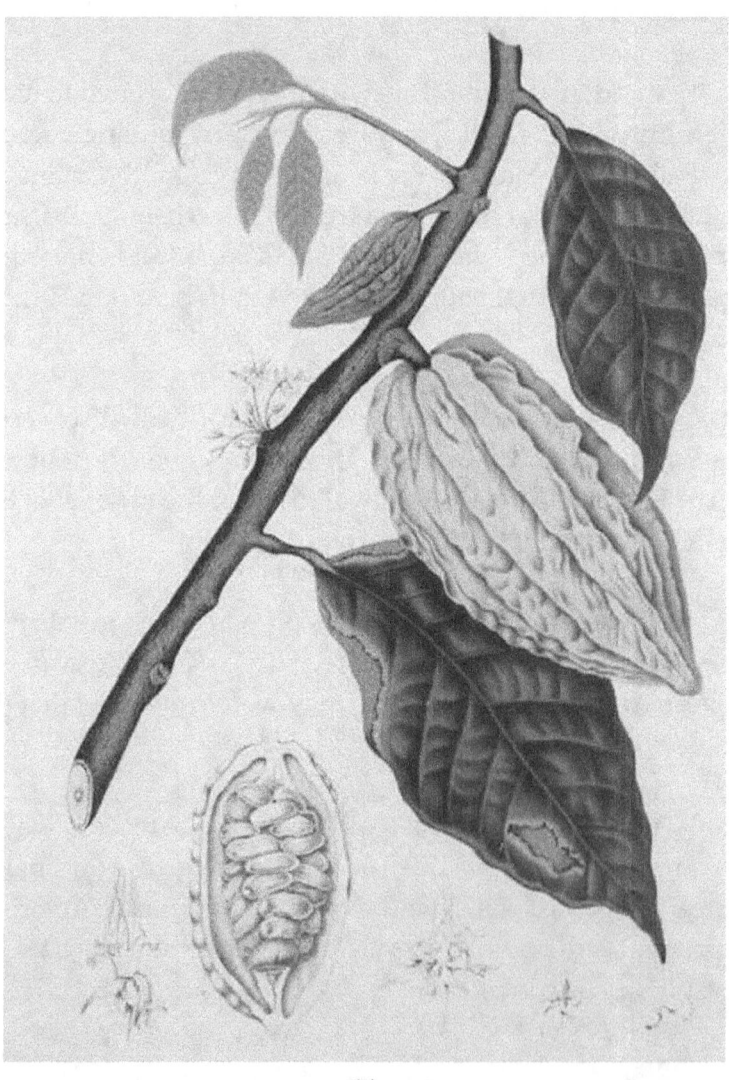

about 40 seeds roughly the size of lima beans. These seeds are fermented inside a sweet pulp, then roasted and ground to make cocoa.

For nearly 4000 years the world has indulged in chocolate; chocolate bars, candy kisses, hot cocoa, chocolate ice-cream and numerous other forms. The idea of a chocolate treat is far from a modern one. The use of chocolate in the New World by the ancient Olmec civilization (1500 BC-500 BC) in Mesoamerican is well documented and the use of chocolate continued on through the time of the Maya and Aztecs before making its trek across to the Old World in the 16th century.

The formulation and serving techniques of the chocolate were somewhat different than today. Mainly consumed as an unheated liquid by the Maya and generally heated by the Aztecs, chocolate was the drink of choice for the elites and with the addition of hot chilies, maize, spices, peanut butter, vanilla and other flavor and texture enhancers, made the chocolate beverage a spicy and sultry drink enjoyed only by those who are able to afford it or by those who are specifically chosen to enjoy its benefits. Over the years, cacao, its components and chocolate in one form or another, have been used in more ways that just as a pleasurable drink. It is known to have healing and preventative properties and has been documented in both ancient and modern medical journals.

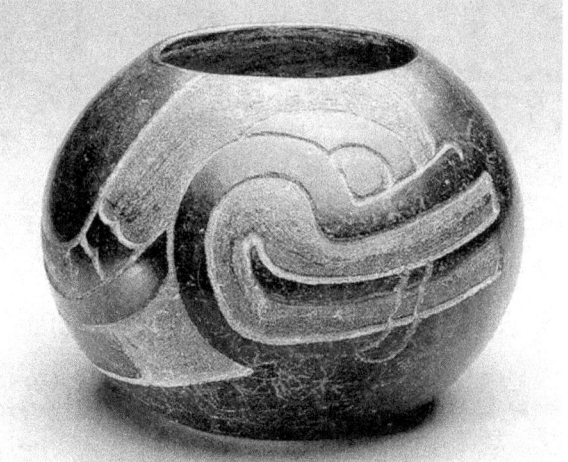

The earliest known use of something we, today, would recognize as chocolate, was by the Olmec peoples around 1900 BC and they enjoyed it as a cold drink and not as a candy bar. The Olmec would drink their chocolate from special round jars known as *tecomates*. Later the Maya would use tall cylinder beakers for drinking their chocolate, and these very often had text on the rim indicating their intended use. The Aztecs also had richly decorated tall cups specifically reserved for chocolate drinks. It may be that conspicuous vessels, such as these, were designed to impress onlookers. To demonstrate or 'show off' that the drinker had the means and status to enjoy such a prized drink. You see, thousands of years ago, only the rich, the powerful, or the warrior class, were able to afford to drink chocolate.

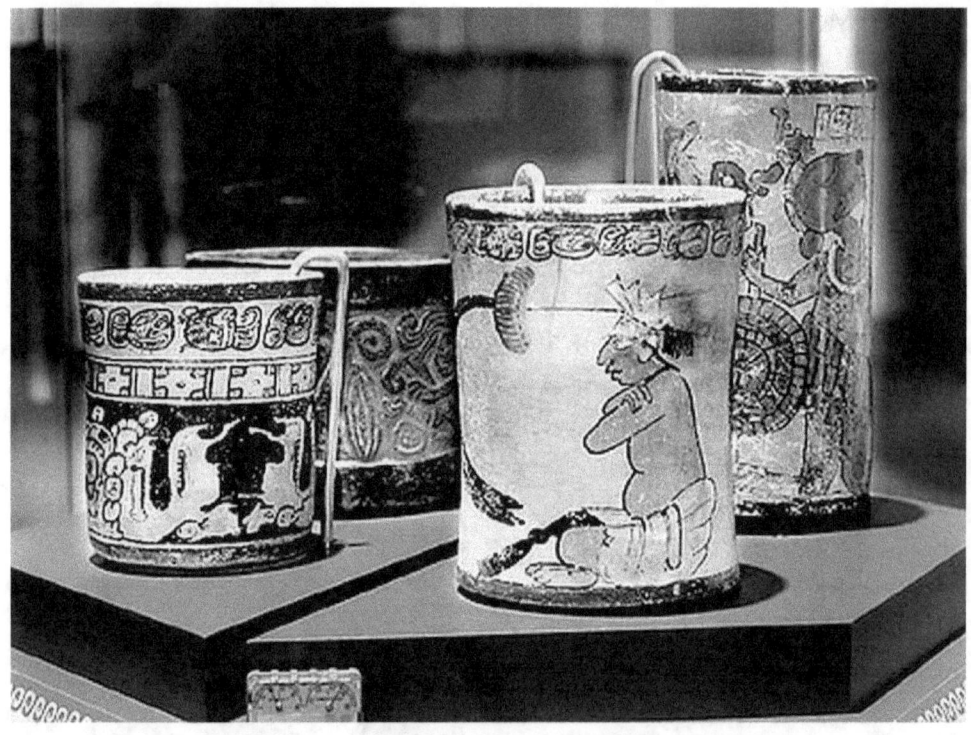

In addition to its loftier role in ritual and celebration, cacao also served decidedly material functions in some early American civilizations. Cocoa beans were kept in locked boxes in businesses, and some enterprising Aztecs actually made counterfeit cocoa beans.

The counterfeits were then passed off as currency or, even more fiendishly, they were hollowed out of their valuable interior and re-filled with a substitute such as sand, and were then passed off as the real thing. At multiple archaeological sites in Mexico and Guatemala, Palka said, researchers have come across quite a number of stashes of remarkably well preserved "cacao beans." "Then they touch them, and it turns out that they are actually not beans at all but are made of clay," he says. The clay beans may have been passed off as money, Palka says, or substituted for real cacao in rituals.

Cocoa quickly became the force of the Aztec economy. The demand for the cocoa bean and the beverage that it produced brought about a huge network of trade routes throughout the region. When the Aztecs conquered the Mayans, they were forced to pay taxes to the Aztecs. These taxes were called "tributes" and they were paid in cocoa, so the Aztecs, who couldn't grow their own cocoa, would always have a supply.

Cacao, like valuables including jadeite and cotton mantles, was commonly exchanged in Maya marriage negotiations at the time of European contact. Chocolate was so esteemed, that the beans were a regularly traded item, very often they were demanded as tribute from subject tribes and the chocolate bean was even used as a form of currency by the Aztecs. As a currency, we know that in Aztec markets one cacao bean could buy you a tomato, 5 beans got you a large pumpkin, 10 beans could get you a woman's company for the night, 30 beans could get you a rabbit and, for the more ambitious shopper, a turkey could be had for 100 beans.

Considering that chocolate was such an expensive item, it comes as no surprise that it was consumed almost exclusively by the upper classes and was usually saved until the end of a meal and then was drunk, typically accompanied by the smoking of another pricey item, tobacco.

Noted archaeologist Eleanor Harrison-Buck, however, cautions against distilling cacao's importance to its economic value as "a form of currency that elites could control and administer as a means of consolidating their power." Rather, she said, the production, acquisition, and circulation of cacao as a resource among the ancient Maya was grounded in social relations.

"I think that chocolate became so important because it's harder to grow," compared to plants like maize and cactus, which were used to brew early versions of beer and tequila, respectively. "You can't grow cacao in every region in the Americas," Palka says. "It requires a certain kind of soil, amount of rainfall, and especially shade because the midges and little flies that pollinate the cacao trees have to live in shade." As a result, cacao requires an area of limited sun and plenty of humidity.

According to archaeologist Harrison-Buck, an official Spanish account from 1618 describes the Belize River town of Lucu, which had "much thick cacao that turns reddish-brown and tastes good by itself." Vanilla vines and annatto trees growing nearby were used to flavor cacao beverages. And art recovered from the Maya Lowlands shows cacao as a staple in ancient Maya feasts. The fact that cacao "served as a key cultigen and staple in ritual feasts for numerous Mesoamerican cultures for thousands of years," Harrison-Buck says, "makes it something particularly important to study and understand in this region."

But the pollen, fossilized plant tissue, and botanical remains of this important crop do not preserve well, she says, in the wet, tropical environments of the Maya Lowlands where cacao was grown and continues to grow today. As a result, archaeologists know more about the early uses of cacao than they do about ancient methods of producing the bean. "There's a lot we still don't know and may never know," Lavis says.

To better understand how ancient civilizations produced cacao, however, Harrison-Buck and soil scientist Serita Frey have been working in Belize to find out whether cacao orchards leave a distinctive biological footprint in soil. Over the past few years, the pair have collected soil in areas where cacao is currently grown in eastern Belize, and begun analyzing it in Frey's lab. They've also sampled soil from floodplains adjacent to ancient Maya sites, and from lands that supported cacao in colonial times.

"We know that when the Spanish arrived in the 16th century, the Maya planted cacao trees right on the riverbanks," says Harrison-Buck. At these humid, biologically diverse sites littered with fallen leaves, the scientists often hear birdsong in the morning. Troops of howler monkeys swing, cry, and feast in fig trees that grow along the river and provide the shade that cacao trees need to thrive.

According to Harrison-Buck, the team has successfully uncovered evidence of a theobromine signature, but the signature is difficult to consistently isolate from older orchard sites. Eventually, by comparing chemicals in soil from these various sites, they're hoping to map out the molecular signposts that indicate ancient cacao cultivation, and reconstruct where cacao was produced in the Belize Valley in historic or even prehistoric times.

There is also some evidence that a lower quality chocolate may have been enjoyed, mixed with a maize gruel by the poorer classes at important events such as weddings, but some scholars maintain that the pure chocolate drink was an exclusive status symbol of the nobility. Curiously, it has been noted by archeologists that their research indicates that chocolate may even have been given to favored sacrificial victims as a final 'purification' before they departed this world, for example, at the annual Aztec festival of Panquetzaliztli held in honor of Huitzilopochtli.

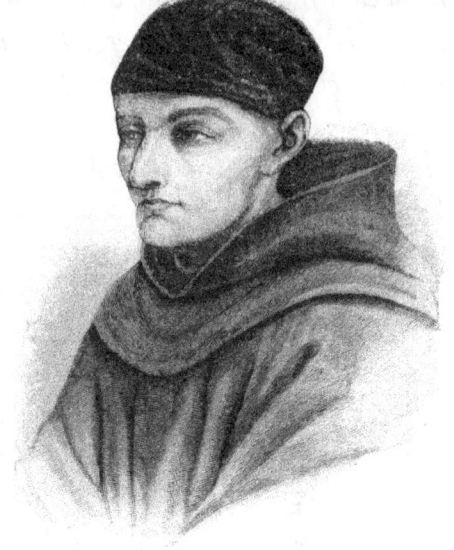

Bernardino de Sahagún (1499 – 1590) who was responsible for writing the _Florentine Codex_, which detailed many Aztec medical practices, was a Franciscan friar, who was sent to the New World as a missionary priest. He is remembered best as a hard working and pioneering Catholic ethnographer who participated in the evangelization of colonial New Spain (known to us today as Mexico). Born in Sahagún, Spain, in 1499, he journeyed to New Spain in 1529. He learned Nahuatl and spent more than 50 years in the study of Aztec beliefs, culture and history. Though he was primarily devoted to his missionary task, his extraordinary work documenting indigenous worldview and culture has earned him the title as "the first anthropologist."

He wrote a vivid eye-witness account of how chocolate was prepared by Aztec women and how to tell a good quality drink from an inferior one:

"...the preparer of fine chocolate is one who grinds, who provides people with drink, and with repasts. She grinds cacao beans; she crushes, breaks, pulverizes them. She chooses, selects, and separates them. She drenches, soaks, and steeps them. She adds water sparingly, conservatively; aerates it, filters it, strains it, pours it back and forth, aerates it; she makes it form a head, makes it foam. She removes the head, makes it form a head again, makes it well foamed... She sells good, superior, potable chocolate: the privilege, the drink of nobles, of rulers - finely ground, soft, foamy, reddish, bitter; with chili water, or with flowers, with uei nacaztli, or with teonacaztli, with vanilla, or with mecaxochitl, with wild bee honey, or with powdered aromatic flowers. Inferior chocolate has maize flour and lime water included; it is pale; the froth bubbles burst."

To prepare the chocolate, cacao beans were fermented, cured, and roasted. Then the beans were ground into powder and mixed with hot water, as chocolate was usually (but not always) consumed as a warm frothy drink, the froth made by vigorously whisking the liquid with a wooden implement and pouring the liquid from one vessel to another. It has been recorded that the froth was considered the best part of the drink. Bitter to taste, it could be flavored by adding, maize, vanilla, flowers, ground chili peppers, herbs, honey, or fermented agave sap (*octli*). Apart from the taste, another advantage of chocolate was that it also contained caffeine and so was used as a stimulant.

Though ancient peoples who consumed cacao were not explicitly aware of its chemical composition, their perpetual use of cacao for medicinal purposes is consistent with the fact that cacao contains these stimulants. The Mayans, for example, equipped warriors with cacao, and as a result were considered invincible and under spiritual protection. In reality, it is likely that the stimulating nature of the alkaloids in cacao were beneficial during battle. The Aztecs also had therapeutic purposes for cacao, in that they believed serving cacao to people before sacrificing them would comfort and purify them.

In addition, in Sahagún's <u>Florentine Codex</u>, the friar described the Aztec cultural and medical practices, with highly detailed information on the various medicinal uses for cacao:

"Chocolate was drunk by the Mexica to treat stomach and intestinal complaints, and when the cacao was combined with liquid from the bark of the silk cotton tree (Castilla elastic), it was said to cure infections."

The medicinal use of cacao occurred in the Old World as well; before modern medicine, treating illness in Europe was based on Galen's system of humors. This system divided diagnoses into hot, wet, cold, and dry, and treated by balancing opposites. Similarly, Aztec medicine also used a method of contrasting treatments, such as hot vs. cold, that was lost in history but picked up on by Europeans. This led to the use of chocolate in European medicine, which could treat sickness differently in its different product forms. For example, native chocolate flavorings were considered "hot" and could warm the stomach to aid in digestion.

Chocolate is often said to have been seen as an ancient medicine and aphrodisiac. Cortez wrote to King Carlos I of Spain of "xocoatl," a drink that "builds up resistance and fights fatigue." And one officer serving Cortez reportedly observed the Aztec ruler Montezuma drinking more than 50 cups per day of a frothy chocolate beverage mixed with water or wine and seasonings including vanilla, pimiento, and chili pepper.

But according to Lavis, some of these tales are likely overstated: "I don't think any living person could drink 50 cups of cacao." The Spanish also probably attributed medical benefits to chocolate that the Maya didn't—instead, cacao was simply part of Mayan life. "I think it was just part of their diet, and they knew it was good for them," Lavis said.

"When you have something that people drink for ritual, people think it's good for you," Palka said. "I would categorize it with eating maize: you have to eat it to sustain your body and yourself and your soul. Chocolate fits clearly into that."

It is believed that it was the Mayan that really brought chocolate into the mainstream considering it as a fully embraced, common, everyday foodstuff. In the 6th century, the Mayan started to use the cocoa bean to make chocolate drinks. Some even think that the word "chocolate" comes from the Maya word *xocoatl*, which means "bitter water." To the Mayas, cocoa pods symbolized life and fertility. Stones from their palaces and temples revealed many craved pictures of cocoa pods. The Maya also used chocolate in religious rituals; it sometimes took the place of blood. Chocolate was used in marriage ceremonies, where it was exchanged by the bride and groom, and in baptisms. They even had a cacao god, Ek Chuah.

The Maya prepared chocolate strictly for drinking. Chocolate history doesn't include solid chocolate until the 1850s. Except for that, the way the Maya prepared chocolate wasn't too much different from the way it's prepared today. The final product could be quite different but the preparation was fairly similar. First, the beans were harvested, fermented, and dried. The beans were then roasted and the shells removed, and the rest was ground into a paste. The paste was mixed with hot water and spices, such as chili, vanilla, annatto, allspice, honey, and flowers. Then the mixture was frothed by pouring it back and forth between two containers. They thought the froth was one of the best parts. It would be scooped off, eaten, and then they would 'froth it up again!" Chocolate was also mixed with corn and water to make a sort of gruel. It was similar to the chocolate and corn drink Pinole, still enjoyed in Latin America today.

With all that was often mixed with the chocolate the warm, liquid drink could be very different from today's hot cocoa, being laden with chili powder and other spices making it a hot and sultry treat popular with royalty while lay people occasionally enjoyed its healing qualities. The Spanish who moved into Mesoamerica were unfamiliar with the 'savage' flavors of the spicy chocolate and determined that it would not be popular as it stood and was not to be sent back home without proper 'adjustments' like the elimination of many of the hot spices and the addition of sweetening ingredients. While archaeological evidence for cacao use by the Aztecs and Maya is rather limited, pictorial and iconographic evidence is quite substantial.

The indigenous peoples of the South American continent used the cacao bean for hundreds of years. Depending on the region of the Americas, certain indigenous groups have documented their use of the cacao back to between 1900 and 300 BC. It is believed that the Olmec tribe was growing trees of cacao, however, the Mayans were the only tribe of the Americas to plant, and maintain, a full-blown cacao plantation, which they did as early as 600 BC. Most researchers note that the cacao trees were growing for thousands of years before its cultivation by humans.

By 1400 AD, the Mayan power was decreasing. The Aztecs ruled over the highlands of central Mexico, far from the rainforests of the Mayans. Since the Aztecs could not grow their own cocoa, they had to trade to get the beans.

The Aztecs also had their own word for chocolate:
chocolatl (cho co LA til), which was very similar to the Mayan word xocolatl. According to Aztec legend, Quetzacoatl (ket za koh AH tul), the Aztec God of Vegetation, came to earth with a cocoa tree and taught the mortals how to cultivate cocoa and make a drink out of its beans. This made the other gods furious, and they threw him out of paradise for

sharing the sacred drink with humans. When he left, he vowed he would return—a promise that would bring about tremendous consequences for the Aztecs.

King Montezuma, the Aztec king, was reported to drink 50 cups of cocoa every day, and an extra one when he was going to meet a lady friend. The drink was so precious that it was often served in golden goblets that were thrown away after just one use!

Unlike the Mayans, drinking cocoa was 100% a luxury in which very few Aztecs were allowed to indulge. Aztecs believed that wisdom and power came from eating the fruit of the cocoa tree. Because of its stimulating effects, however, Aztec women were forbidden to drink it. You don't want a bunch of over stimulated women running around, filled with power and wisdom, I suppose, they might just band together and take over!

Before chocolate covered strawberries, had sea salt sprinkled on top, or was a sticky topping on ice cream it was a crop that originated in the New World particularly the central and southern part of the Americas. The cacao, was not given the name cacao until European settlers arrived. Although, Mayan scripts have reference to such substance as kawkaw. The genus name for the plant was not given until a European scientist named it. However, the actual word "chocolate" is very similar to the Aztect word xocolatl and may have been pronounced very close to the way we pronounce chocolate today.

Upon Columbus' arrival in 1492, he was greeted many indigenous peoples and was given many gifts by them. One, no doubt, was chocolate and he is credited as the first European to have encountered the cocoa bean. Doing so within just a few short years into his stay. Between the years of 1502 and 1504 during Columbus' fourth voyage from the Americas', he is known to have brought Cacao beans back with him to Europe. According to his own reports he stumbled onto a canoe full of a variety of foods and the cacao seeds were one of many things he found. Learning of the

"Indian's" fondness for chocolate beans, he took them back with him to Europe. When he returned to Spain, he brought some cocoa beans back to the court of King Ferdinand and Queen Isabella, but they were not especially interested in the strange new bean. In the 1500s, Cortes is also noted to have brought cacao beans from Mexico. Taking them across the Atlantic Ocean back again, to the king of Spain. He, and other conquerors helped to spread the cacao bean to other places in the world. It eventually became a favorite of the King, who used it to flavor his 'not so pure' water.

Hernan Cortes first arrived in the Aztec homeland in 1519, the same year Quetzacoatl had promised to return. Cortes happened to land at the exact spot from which the Aztec god departed. In his feather coated armor and gold jewelry, he reminded Aztecs of their returning god. No wonder Montezuma offered him a cup of cocoa and an entire cocoa plantation! It made Cortes' conquest of the Aztec empire all the easier.

The history of chocolate in Spain is part of the culinary history of the country as understood since the 16th century, when the colonization of the Americas began and the cocoa plant was discovered in regions of Mesoamerica. That culinary history continues right up to the present.

After the conquest of Mexico, cocoa as a commodity, travelled by ship from the port of Nueva España across the Atlantic to the Spanish coast. The first such voyage to Europe occurred at an unknown date in the 1520s. However, it was only in the 17th century that regular trade began from the port of Veracruz, opening a maritime trade route that would supply the new demand from Spain, and later from other European countries.

The introduction of this ingredient in Spanish culinary traditions was immediate, compared with other ingredients brought from Latin America, and its popularity and acceptance in all sectors of Spanish society reached very high levels by the end of the 16th century. Since its inception, chocolate was considered by Spaniards as a drink, just as it had been used in the New World. It retained that perception until the beginning of the 20th century.

From the early stages, the cocoa was sweetened with sugar cane, which the Spanish were the first to popularize in Europe. In pre-Columbus America chocolate was flavored with peppers, herbs, and spices and was a mixture of both bitter and spicy flavors. This made it an acquired taste and limited its appeal to the Spanish conquistadors, who were soon encouraged to sweeten it with sugar brought from the Iberian Peninsula. Cortes did not enjoy the bitter cocoa drink, but he was amazed at how the Aztecs valued it. The brilliant solution Cortes came up with: mix the drink with copious amounts of honey or cane sugar and serve it hot. Cortes described the resulting mixture as "the divine drink which builds up resistance and fights fatigue," As a result, his men than began consuming it heated too, rather than cold, and "hot chocolate" was born.

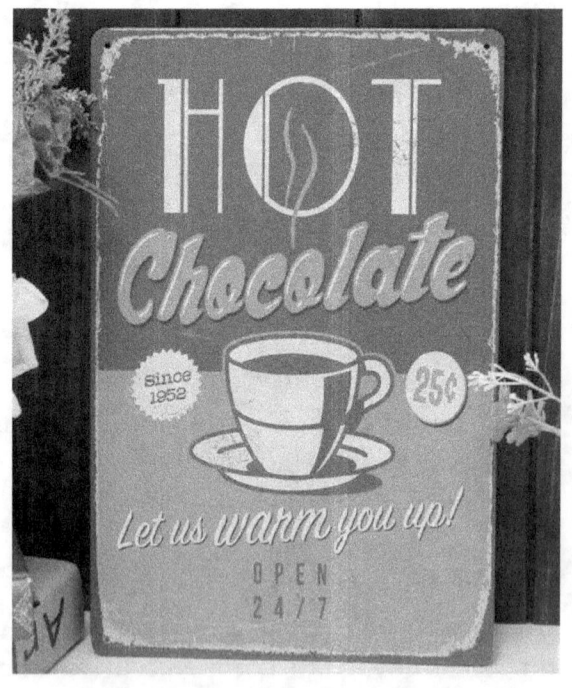

July 7th was an important day back in the 16th century. It was Chocolate Day, the observance of the date in 1550 when chocolate was introduced to Europe from the New World. The date is certainly questionable, since

Christopher Columbus presented cacao beans (the source of chocolate) decades earlier to King Ferdinand and Queen Isabella. The beans, however, were apparently no more than a curiosity until Hernando Cortes made improvements to Aztec chocolate. In 1519, the Aztecs had welcomed Cortes with the offering of a liquid chocolate, unsweetened, beverage that one conquistador described as "a bitter drink for pigs."

I mentioned earlier that the King and Queen of Spain did not like the chocolate that they first encountered. But when Cortes returned to Spain in 1528, the King and Queen took notice. You see, unlike Columbus, years earlier, Cortes brought not only the beans but the recipe and the equipment necessary to make the chocolate beverage. For several decades, cocoa was mostly a Spanish secret, but then its popularity quickly spread to the other countries of Europe

Over a 100-year period since its first appearance in the ports of Andalusia, chocolate became popular as a drink in Spain, where it was served to the Spanish monarchy. However, for a time the formula was unknown in the rest of Europe. Okay, I say unknown, but the truth is that the Spanish kept the cocoa beans secret from the rest of Europe for a long time. In 1579, English pirates attacked a Spanish merchant ship filled with cocoa beans. Thinking the beans were dried sheep droppings, the pirates burned the ship in frustration. Some say the first chocolate makers were actually monks hidden away in monasteries who mistakenly shared their "secret" with their French counterparts.

Whatever the case, once cocoa started catching on, Spanish cooks experimented with the recipe and added sugar to sweeten it. That did it! Chocolate was here to stay, once the cocoa caught on, it caught on big. Like the Mayans and Aztecs, the Spanish drank cocoa for health and energy. But they also enjoyed it during church services and were even allowed to have cocoa during Lent, because it was considered a necessary beverage.

The great popularity of the drink in Spanish society from its introduction until the 19th century was attested to in various reports written by travelers who visited the Iberian Peninsula. It was said that "chocolate is to the Spanish what tea is to the English". In this way chocolate was converted into a national symbol. The unusual fondness for this drink meant that coffee remained relatively unpopular in Spain compared to other European countries. In Spain, chocolate was exclusively considered a refreshing drink, and it was rarely used in other ways—though there are older Spanish dishes that use cocoa. After the Spanish Civil War (1936 to 1939) the custom declined in favor of coffee consumption. In modern Spain, traces of the history of the drink can be seen in the chocolate companies, the chocolate shops and museums.

Later chocolate spread from Spain to Portugal, France, Italy, Germany, Holland and England. The first countries outside of Spain, to embrace chocolate were Italy, France and Belgium.

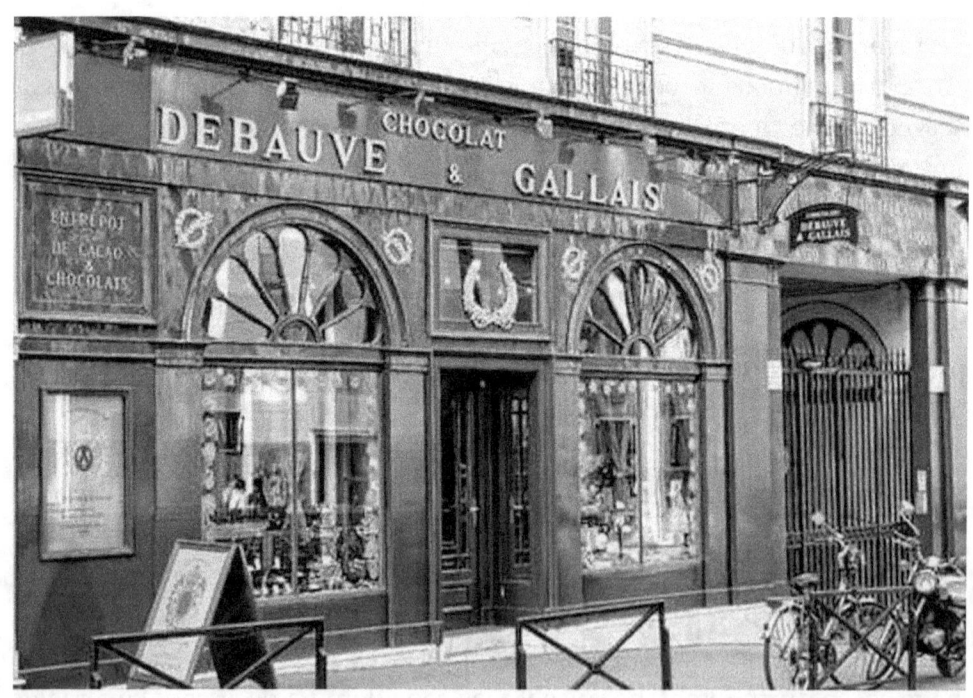

In 1615, cocoa found its way into the court of the King Louis the Thirteenth of France at his royal wedding. King Louis Thirteenth married the Spanish princess Anne d'Autriche. Anne not only brought cocoa along in her wedding basket, she also brought a servant skilled in the art of making the foaming beverage. Their son, Louis the Fourteenth, was not a great cocoa fancier, but he played a major role in popularizing the drink. In 1659, he granted David Chaillou a 'royal authorization' to open the first chocolaterie in Paris. Chaillou roasted the beans in a pan and ground them the same way the Mayans and the Aztecs did, but that was about to change.

Although the Spanish had actually brought chocolate back to Europe in the late 1500s – early 1600s they were essentially able to keep it secret for nearly a century. In 1667, a Frenchman opened the first chocolate house in London. It was called _The Coffee Mill and The Tobacco Roll_, and because of the cost of the drink, only upper class could buy 'Chocolate water.' But due to the popularity of chocolate drink, it started to make an appearance as an ingredient in cakes and rolls as early as 1674. Because the drink was still considered a luxury, the shops were only open to men as a place to gamble and discuss politics.

Up until the mid-1700s, chocolate was made much the same way the ancient Mayans made it. Then during the industrial revolution, a series of technological innovations changed many things including the way chocolate was made. First, a Frenchman named Doret invented a hydraulic machine to grind cocoa beans into paste. Soon after, another Frenchman named Dubuisson created a steam driven chocolate mill.

After Great Britain's first chocolate manufacturing plant opened in 1730, a huge candy industry based itself on the irresistible flavor: Mints. Nougats. Bars. Truffles. Drinks. Cakes and frostings. To adapt a famous advertising slogan, "Without chocolate, life itself would be impossible."

Chocolate soothed egos, stimulated ids, and put Hershey, Pa., on the map. It entered the culture as a lover's gift. In the old world, as in the new, it reached almost religious status: Carolus Linnaeus, who originated scientific naming of species, called the tree Theobroma cacao. Theobroma translates as "food of the gods."

In 1847, Joseph Fry of Bristol, England, made the next major leap, with an improved steam engine for grinding the beans. It was now possible to grind huge amounts of cocoa and mass-produce chocolate inexpensively and quickly so it was available to people all over Europe. Chocolate was no longer reserved for the elite.

The steam engine was crucial in mechanizing the process of grinding cacao seeds to produce chocolate. Before the steam engine, cacao seeds were ground in mills driven by animal, wind, or water power, and before that they were ground by hand with stones. The power supplied by the steam engine enabled chocolate makers to streamline chocolate production in larger quantities.

Before Fry & Sons could create the chocolate bar, however, a Dutch chemist, Coenraad Van Houten, invented the cocoa press in 1829. It squeezed the cocoa butter out of the bean leaving the powder we now call cocoa. He also added alkaline salts to powdered chocolate, which helps it mix better with water, and gives it a darker color and milder flavor. This process is called "dutching" after the nationality of the inventor. All of these innovations made chocolate smoother, creamier and tastier.

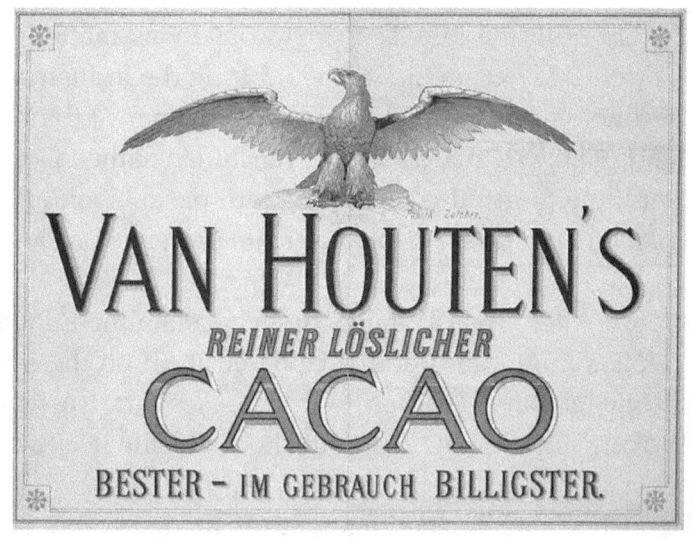

How important was the cocoa press? Van Houten's invention made it possible to separate the dry part of the cocoa bean (cocoa powder) and the wet part of the bean (cocoa butter). This separation now allowed chocolatiers to add different amounts of cocoa butter and cocoa powder together to make various flavors of chocolate. Without the cocoa press, we would not have white chocolate, milk chocolate or cocoa powder for making hot cocoa and baking

In 1830, Swiss Chocolatier Charles-Amedee Kohler mixed chocolate with nuts for the first time. But a truly revolutionary advance occurred in 1847, when the Fry Company of Bristol, England created the world's first eating chocolate. One year later, the very first chocolate bar appeared. After a 1000-year history as a beverage, this was the first-time chocolate could be eaten!

Then, in 1875, Swiss born Daniel Peter (son-in-law of Henri Nestlé) added condensed milk to chocolate…thereby creating the first 'milk chocolate.' The food of the gods had come a long way from the spicy, bitter brew the Mayans knew.

In today's more health-conscious society though we're seeing a health trend back to the dark chocolate with a higher cacao content and more bitter taste. It is estimated that the average American eats at least a half a pound of chocolate, dark or light, sweet, or a little more bitter, each and every month. This American must admit that he probably exceeds that!

In 1879, Rodolphe Lindt created the conching machine, which ground the gritty, chocolate paste into a rich, smooth blend. Around 1900, an "enrobing" machine replaced the task of hand dipping all of the chocolates.

In 1895, Jean Neuhaus began wrapping nuts with chocolate. In 1912, he perfected the technique of molded chocolates, or pralines, by adding fillings inside a chocolate shell. In Belgium, pralines filled with creams, ganaches, and marzipans were so successful that a new box had to be created. The "ballotin," which is the French word for "gift box," was designed to keep the precious pralines from breaking. It is from this that we derive the word valentine.

2. Belgium & Swiss Chocolate

Several years ago, I read somewhere about an order of Mexican nuns who became so besotted with chocolate that they neglected their work, their works of charity, and worst of all, their prayer life. Morning, noon, and night, life revolved around making and consuming chocolate. Eventually, the Holy Father himself sanctioned them by imposing a lifetime ban on the consumption of chocolate in that convent. That just goes to show how much we all love chocolate – especially in Belgium and Switzerland!

Belgium

One can hardly talk about the history of chocolate without bringing Belgium into the conversation – that would be like talking about beer without mentioning Germany (shameless plug there – my next book will be about the history and health benefits of Beer!)

Chocolate much like fashion, wine and finance, has become a complex cultural phenomenon. There is basic chocolate for the masses, artisanal chocolate for purists and avant-garde creations for connoisseurs. In Brussels, a polyglot city at the geographic and cultural crossroads of Europe, you get it all.

The capital of Belgium may be known as the Capital of Europe, but it is also, at least as far as most chocolate aficionados are concerned, the World Capital of Chocolate. Ever since the Brussels chocolatier Jean Neuhaus invented the praline 100 years ago, the city has been at the forefront of the chocolate business. There are a million residents and some 500 chocolatiers, about one chocolatier for every 2,000 people. The average Belgian consumes over 15 pounds of chocolate each year, one of the highest rates in the world.

But these days, the industry is changing. With countries like Germany and the Netherlands becoming larger European exporters, in Belgium, a new class of chocolatiers is finding innovative ways to hold on to the country's chocolate crown. They are breaking away from traditional pralines — which Belgians classify as any chocolate shell filled with a soft fondant center — and infusing ganaches with exotic flavors like wasabi or lemon verbena, and creating such imaginative pairings as blackcurrant and cardamom and raspberry and clove.

If you find yourself in Brussels, intent on exploring three centuries of chocolate history, I hope you give yourself plenty of time. It is an ambitious task: the city is home to two of the biggest chocolate companies in the world, Godiva and Leonidas, as well as scores of boutique chocolate-makers and haute chocolatiers.

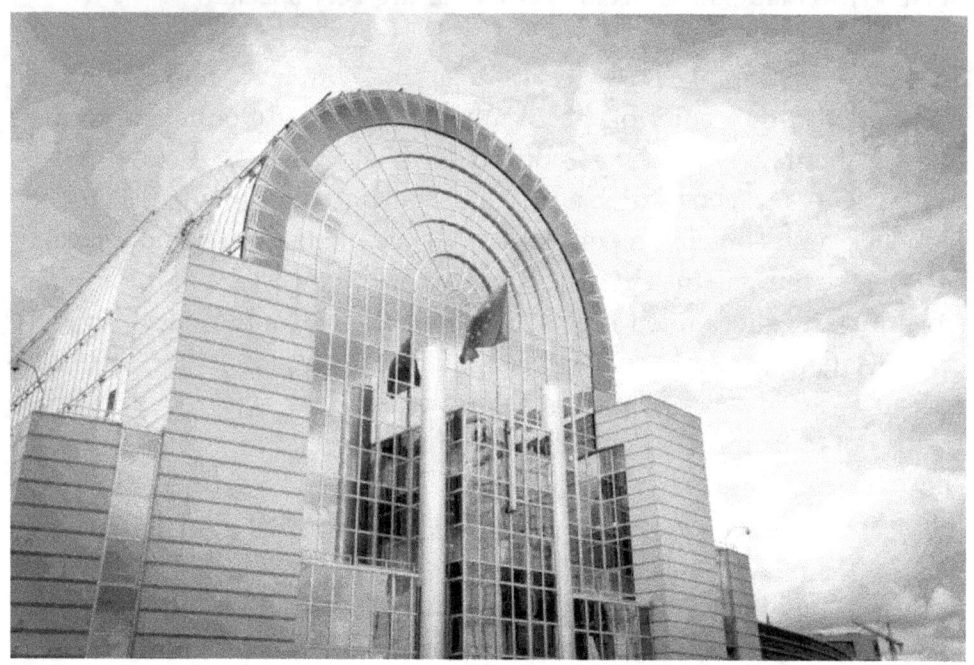

Brussels is a curious mix of conservative and avant-garde — in the European quarter alone, you have the cylinder-shaped glass dome of the European Parliament's Paul-Henri Spaak building hovering over the neo-Classical-style Place du Luxembourg, while graffito-studded beacons of

Art Nouveau architecture reside nearby. The city's chocolate scene reflects that tension. The result is some wonderfully surprising creations. To get a real sense of it, I turned to Robbin Zeff Warner, an American expatriate and a former professor of writing at George Washington University who has been blogging about Belgian chocolatiers since her husband's post with NATO took them to Brussels in 2008.

"You have chocolate for tourists, and chocolate for Belgians," Ms. Warner said of the national hierarchy in which chocolate produced by manufacturers like Côte d'Or and Guylian are devoured in vast quantities, but mostly by the city's six million annual visitors. Bruxellois, Ms. Warner said, prefer the artisanal makers. "The big-name big houses are great. But seeing and tasting real handmade chocolate, while buying it from the person who made the chocolate, is something very special."

To prove her point, I suggest a visit to Wittamer, the century-old chocolatier in the center of the city that seduces both locals and tourists with its heritage recipes, or you could go to Alex & Alex, a nearby Champagne and chocolate bar. Though its chocolates, made by Frederic Blondeel, aren't made on-site, they're acknowledged in some circles as some of the finest in the city. The bar is tucked away on one of the antiques store-and art gallery-filled streets that shoot off the Grand Sablon, Brussels' central square. Its dark, cozy interior, along with a glass of Drappier rosé and an array of square bonbons before you, well, it is just an experience that is not to be missed in this lifetime. I recommend the "Alex'Perience" chocolates - that first velvety impression of high-quality chocolate, followed by a flood of sweet, fruity cassis is unworldly!

Spend the afternoon circling the Grand Sablon, which, with no fewer than eight chocolatiers, is the city's epicenter of chocolate. You can sample golf-ball-size truffles at Godiva and molded hamster heads at Leonidas; organic nougat from Pure and minty ganaches at Passion. At Neuhaus, try a dark chocolate truffle filled with buttercream and with speculoos, a spicy Belgian cookie. After all of this you will understand why chocolate aficionados the world over call Belgium, the World Capital of Chocolate.

The more one strolls, the clearer it will become that the level of sophistication is still evolving. The packaging and presentation at newer chocolatiers is as slick as a Place Vendôme showroom, while the associated terminology — like "cru" and "domain" — is akin to what you'd hear from sommeliers discussing the finest wines. Such is the case at Pierre Marcolini's two-story flagship. Smiling sales people stand over glassed-in displays of small, rectangular bonbons that look as exquisite as jewels. Backlighted shelves on the opposite wall showcased what Mr. Marcolini is famous for: his single-origin Grand Cru chocolate bars. A must have item!

Over a dozen years ago, in 2004, Mr. Marcolini raised the bar when he started scouting the globe for the best cocoa beans. He became the only chocolatier in Brussels to work directly with plantations in countries like Venezuela and Madagascar, bringing the beans back to his ateliers for roasting and grinding. "Most people think it's the percentage that makes a difference," said a saleswoman, speaking of the amount of cocoa in the confections, "but it's the origin of the cocoa bean that does. It's a little bit like wine." Indeed, when you bite into the Cuban cru — Marcolini claims to be the only chocolatier in the world working with cacao from Cuba — you will detect vibrant notes of dried cherries in the slightly acidic chocolate.

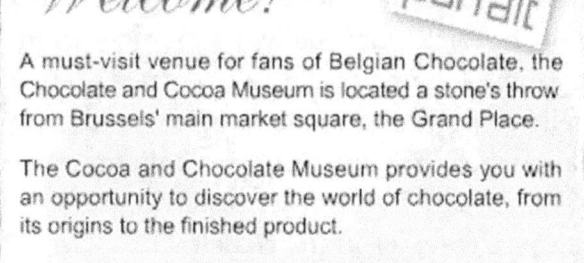

Welcome! Un diner presque parfait

A must-visit venue for fans of Belgian Chocolate, the Chocolate and Cocoa Museum is located a stone's throw from Brussels' main market square, the Grand Place.

The Cocoa and Chocolate Museum provides you with an opportunity to discover the world of chocolate, from its origins to the finished product.

Step into the history of the Aztecs and the Mayas, who used to grow cocoa thousands of years ago. You will also discover how cocoa finally ended up in Europe.
The various posters, video presentations and display panels available in the Museum are designed to show you how cocoa is grown and processed into chocolate.

The highlight of the visit is a demonstration given by a master chocolate maker showing how pralines are made in a traditional way.

Another 'chocolate stop' while in Brussels has to be the 300+ year-old Museum of Cocoa and Chocolate:

Back in the 17th century, when Belgium was still ruled by the Spanish, explorers brought cocoa beans from South America and introduced them to the Belgian community. At the time, chocolate was a sign of luxury and was mostly used to make 'hot chocolate' for nobility or to impress new visitors. In fact, Henri Escher, the major of Zurich, was served a cup of this delicious drink when visiting the Grand Place of Brussels in 1697. He immediately fell in love with it, took the recipe home with him, and introduced his own country to chocolate. Switzerland is now considered Belgium's biggest competitor regarding the production and distribution of chocolates.

As we all know however, chocolate is no longer exclusive to the rich and famous — though it may taste exquisitely good, anyone can afford it nowadays. The first-time Belgium truly delved into the chocolate market was when they colonized the Congo and found a large surplus of cocoa beans. King Leopold the Third then made Belgium the number one trader in cocoa and chocolate.

It was Jean Neuhaus (ironically, from Switzerland) who first put Belgian chocolate on the map. In 1857, he moved into a pharmacy-cum-sweet shop in the Galérie de la Reine in Brussels, where he sold plaques of dark chocolate. Gradually, the apothecary transformed into a real sweet shop, and the first praline was created there in 1912. The hollow chocolate shell with a sweet filling was invented by Jean's grandson (also named Jean) who also invented the Ballotin, the box in which pralines are wrapped. The Jean Neuhaus store still exists to this day, and is deemed a must-see when visiting Brussels.

To understand why Belgian chocolates are so famous and deliciously addictive, it is important to know exactly how they are made. The secret to their success lies in the ingredients used to make them and, of course, in the production process. A law created in 1884 states that a minimum level of 35% cocoa must be used, in order to prevent the usage of low-quality fat sources or other 'hacks' to modify the composition. Production starts in the early stages, which includes overseeing how the cocoa beans are planted, the way they are roasted, and which beans are used.

There are several laws and unspoken rules in the chocolate-making community, where traditional manufacturing is preferred. This explains why there are so many small, independent chocolatiers throughout Belgium. However, even big chocolatiers like Neuhaus have managed to expand outside Belgium, but still continue to use only traditional recipes for their chocolates, many of which are still held even more "top secret" than the Coronel's 11 herbs and spices.

As I mentioned above, if you're in Belgium and want to learn about the chocolate-making process in more detail, it is worth visiting the Museum of Cocoa and Chocolate, the MUCC, which is located near the Grand Place, Brussels' main market square. A new 'game' the museum came up with, the Truck game, allows you to walk through the city center of Brussels while discovering the world of chocolate within the city.

The best known commercial brand of Belgian chocolate is Côte d'Or, which you can find in almost any grocery store in Belgium and in many places around the world. Côte d'Or was founded by Charles Neuhaus in 1870, who opened a factory shortly after that. The name refers to the Golden Coast, now Ghana in Africa, where the cocoa beans first originated from. The brand is now part of the American multinational company Mondelez International, whose other products include Oreo, Toblerone, Mikado, Milka, and Cadbury.

Commercial brands such as Neuhaus are renowned for making delicious chocolates, and their regular chocolate bars, pralines and truffles are definitely a must try when visiting Belgium — but the products of local, independent chocolatiers are certainly worth sampling as well!

Today, Belgian chocolate is world-renowned and continues to play a strong role in the Belgian economy. Overall, there are over 2,000 chocolatiers in the country, so anyone who visits Belgium shouldn't hesitate to try this delicious treat. As you can tell I am partial to Belgium chocolate but we really cannot talk about chocolate in Europe with mentioning the chocolate of Switzerland.

The Swiss

Although Switzerland never colonized any cocoa growing countries like Ghana in Africa or some south American country, they still manage to produce some of the world's leading Chocolate, it is hard to understand how Switzerland manages this amazing feat, but no one can deny that Swiss chocolate is famous world over.

Chocolate was first introduced in Switzerland in 1697 when the mayor of Zurich brought it home after having a chocolate drink in Belgium. At this time, chocolate was a fashionable drink mostly for the aristocracy at parties.

If you mention Switzerland to anyone they are likely to start thinking of cheese, watches and some of the best chocolate in the world! Not surprising as chocolate has been more than just a sweet temptation in Switzerland for more than 200 years. Selected ingredients are blended together in Swiss chocolate. Behind the refined exterior, these are the factors behind the success story of Switzerland: inventive spirit, quality consciousness, hard work – and an uninhibited sense of taste and enjoyment.

However, chocolate does not by any means have its origin in the heart of Europe. The cocoa bean even less so. It was the Aztecs: They drank hot chocolate as early as the 14th century. It is said to have been bitter, even spicy. At any rate, that was the opinion of Hernán Cortés. Nevertheless, he brought cocoa across the Atlantic; the year was around 1520. Soon afterwards, the coffee was refined at the Spanish royal court. Honey, sugar, vanilla and cinnamon make the drink sweeter, milder. But the common people did not even know it by name.

Chocolate then came to the other European courts. And it did so – yes! – thanks to love. When Anna, Princess of Spain, married the French king Louis XIII, chocolate reached France. Great joy in Versailles! It then arrived in no time at all at every royal court in Europe. And every self-respecting person drank chocolate. And that brought the chocolate pioneers onto the scene. There had to be more to this noble commodity! A dessert maybe? Chocolate was not yet available in solid form. They experimented, roasted, ground, mixed: the taste pioneers in Italy, Belgium, Germany, Holland – and particularly in Switzerland.

In the 19th century, a time some in the world of chocolate call "The age of pioneers'" factories were built, the steam engine was invented, the railway, the telephone – and chocolate, soft and melt-in-the-mouth, as we know and love it today. Its inventor: Rodolphe Lindt.

Switzerland, the land of chocolate? In actual fact, the Swiss make chocolate for the whole world. And for themselves: They eat more of it than anyone else.

Small, impassable, and poor, that was Switzerland at the start of the 19th century. Not a very good basis for chocolate experimentalists. It meant that even more enthusiasm, wealth of ideas and entrepreneurial spirit were required. Switzerland had plenty of that and the success story could begin.

From 1819 onwards, the names started to appear that still symbolize Swiss "quality chocolate" today. François-Louis Cailler, founder of the first mechanized chocolate production facility; this was where milk chocolate was invented. Callier chocolate is still a very loved brand today and is now located in Borc and is open to visitors where you can enjoy a grand tour of the factory and eat chocolates of high quality.

Then there was Philippe Suchard, a confectioner of some renown and from 1826 onwards also a chocolate manufacturer; Rudolf Sprüngli-Ammann, founder of the first chocolate production facility in German-speaking Switzerland in came along in 1845. Aquilino Maestrani, a Ticinobased chocolate maker who opened a production facility in Lucerne in 1852 and, of course, there were Jean Tobler and Rodolphe Lindt.

With his chocolat fondant, Rodolphe Lindt laid the foundation of a corperate empire in 1879. He would achieve incredible success with his company, Lindt & Sprüngli AG, which was founded twenty years later, together with Rudolf Sprüngli.

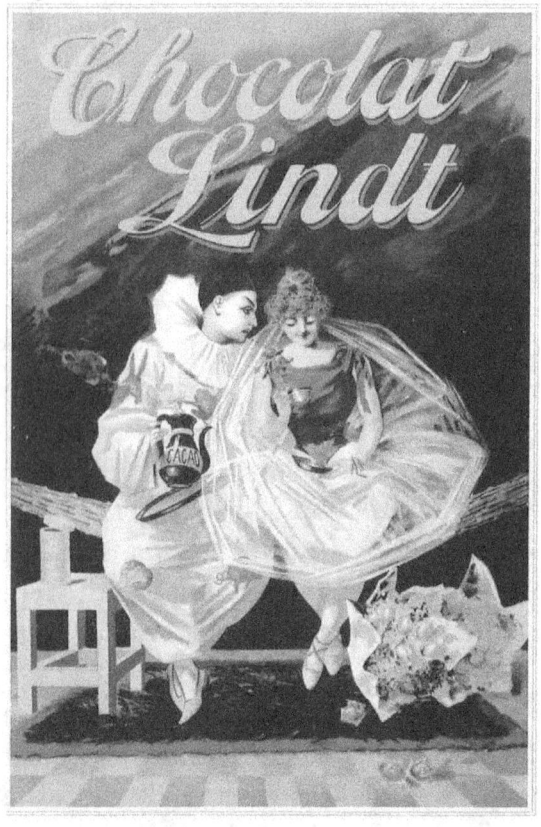

In 1899, Jean Tobler started a chocolate factory in Berne, Tobler originally sold chocolate from Lindt and his own confectionary at his shop.
Later, Mr. Tobler started producing his own unique milk chocolate made with Almonds, nougat and honey.

It is believed that Mr. Tobler got his inspiration of the Toblerone Chocolate from the Matterhorn shape which is triangular, the same shape as the Toblerone candy.

From the year 1890, Switzerland's chocolate industry was already booming and Swiss chocolate was known, not only in Switzerland but abroad. By 1905, Switzerland was already producing 13 tons of chocolate which was considered quite a lot at the time, but by 1918, the production was 40,000 tons, most of it for export.

During the depression years of the 1920s and 1930s, export of Swiss suffered a bit but chocolate sales picked up again, in an incredible way, after the 2nd world war.

In the past, competition among chocolatiers has forced Swiss chocolate producers to streamline production while still improving the quality and reputation. Tradition and quality still remain key sales factors for Swiss chocolate, even today.

Thanks to its unsurpassable quality – and thanks to the growing interest in travel. The English, Germans, Russians and Americans visited Switzerland in droves. Mountains were suddenly très chic. And lakes too. Not to mention hospitality. And what did they take back with them? Chocolat fondant from LINDT and the obligatory Toblerone of course!

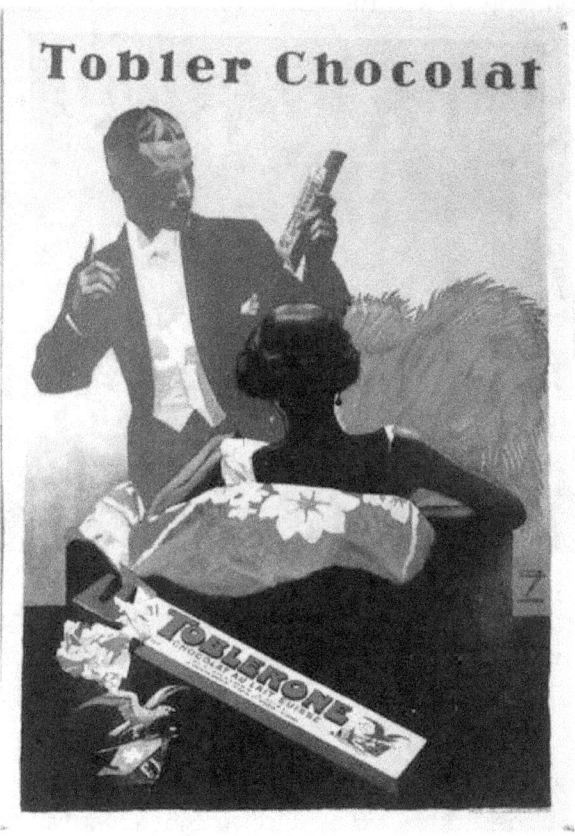

A lot has changed since then. And yet: Rodolphe Lindt's chocolat Surfin is still produced today based on the 1879 recipe and packed in the original wrapping. And the Toblerone? Well, Today Toblerone is the most famous chocolate in all the world.

3. The Chocolate Chip Cookie

Although originally it came from the America's, chocolate had to go to Europe before it was successfully reintroduced to the New World. Almost as an accident chocolate was brought along with English colonists and was 're-established', so to speak, in America. Among my favorite American contributions to the world of chocolate is the chocolate chip cookie.

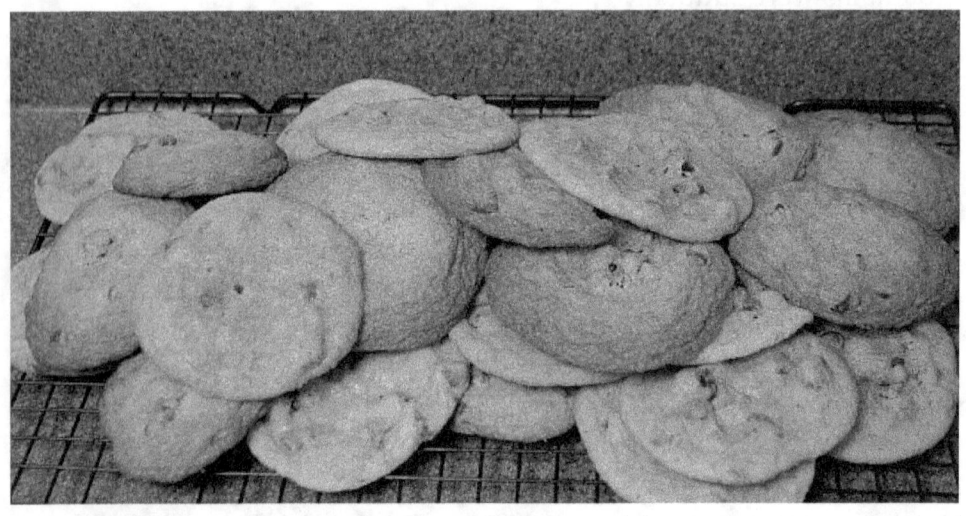

Like chocolate itself, the chocolate chip cookie was also an accident. The chocolate-chip cookie will celebrate its eightieth birthday next year. Unlike the anonymous inventors of such American staples as the hot dog, the grilled-cheese sandwich, and the milkshake, the creator of the chocolate-chip cookie has always been known to us. Ruth Wakefield, who ran the popular Toll House Inn restaurant in Whitman, Massachusetts, with her husband, Kenneth, from 1930 to 1967, brought the Toll House Chocolate Crunch Cookie into being in the late nineteen-thirties. The recipe, which has been tweaked over the ensuing decades, made its first appearance in print in the 1938 edition of Wakefield's "Tried and True" cookbook. Created as an accompaniment to ice cream, the chocolate-chip cookie quickly became so celebrated that Marjorie Husted (a.k.a. Betty

Crocker) featured it on her radio program. As the new chocolate chip cookie's popularity soared, so did sales of the Nestle semi-sweet chocolate bar used in the cookies, and eventually, On March 20, 1939, Ruth Wakefield and Nestle reached an agreement that allowed the company to print the Toll House cookie recipe on the label of Nestle's semi-sweet chocolate bar. In a bargain that rivals Peter Minuit's purchase of Manhattan, the price was a dollar—a dollar that Wakefield later said she never received (though she was reportedly given free chocolate for life and was also paid by Nestlé for work as a consultant).

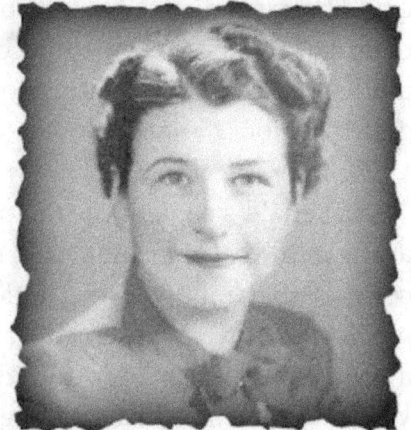

While we have always known the who, the where, and the when of the chocolate-chip cookie's origins, the how and the why have remained somewhat obscure. A set of often-repeated creation myths have grown up around the country's favorite baked good. The most frequently reproduced story is that Wakefield unexpectedly ran out of nuts for a regular ice-cream cookie recipe and, in desperation, replaced them with chunks chopped out of a bar of Nestle #233 bittersweet chocolate. (A variation of this tale has Wakefield substituting the chips after running out of bakers' chocolate.) Another even more unlikely story posits that the vibrations from an industrial mixer caused chocolate stored on a shelf in the Toll House kitchen to fall into a vat of cookie dough as it was being mixed.

None of these, it appears, is true. In her recently published *"Great American Chocolate Chip Cookie Book,"* the food writer Carolyn Wyman offers a more believable, if somewhat less enchanted, telling. Wyman argues, persuasively, that Wakefield, who was a nutritionist with a degree in household arts and a reputation for perfectionism, would not have allowed her restaurant, which was famed for its desserts, to run out of such essential ingredients as bakers' chocolate or nuts. Rather, the more plausible explanation is that Wakefield developed the chocolate-chip cookie "by dint of training, talent, [and] hard work." As prepared as she was, though, it is unlikely that the diligent proprietor of the Toll House Inn could have predicted that her combination of butter, flour, sugar, nuts, and chocolate would go on to become an iconic American food, adored by adults and children, creating fortunes and spawning countless imitations and variations.

Wakefield's cookie was the perfect antidote to the Great Depression. In a single inexpensive hand-held serving, it contained the very richness and comfort that millions of people were forced to live without in the late nineteen-thirties. Ingesting a warm chocolate-chip cookie offered the eaters a brief respite from their quotidian woe. America's entry into the Second World War only enhanced the popularity of Wakefield's creation. Toll House cookies were a common constituent in care packages shipped to American soldiers overseas. Though chocolate was in short supply domestically because of the war effort, women on the home front were encouraged to use what little they had to bake cookies for "that soldier boy of yours," as one Nestlé ad put it. The Toll House restaurant's gift shop alone sent thousands of cookies to uniformed servicemen abroad. "Like Spam and Coca-Cola," Wyman writes, "chocolate chip cookies' fame was boosted by wartime soldier consumption. Before the war, they were a largely East Coast-based fad, but after the war Toll House cookies rivaled apple pie as the most popular dessert recipe in the country."

In the postwar years, the chocolate-chip cookie followed the path taken by many American culinary innovations: from homemade to mass-produced, from kitchen counter to factory floor, from fresh to franchised. In the nineteen-fifties, both Nestlé and Pillsbury began selling refrigerated chocolate-chip-cookie dough in supermarkets. Nabisco, meanwhile, launched Chips Ahoy, its line of packaged cookies, in 1963. The Baby Boom generation, which had been raised on the Toll House cookie, sought to recapture the original taste of these homemade treats in stores that sold fresh-baked cookies. Famous Amos, Mrs. Fields, and David's Cookies all opened their first stores in the seventies, and prospered in the eighties. By the middle of that decade, there were more than twelve hundred cookie stands in business across the country.

The story of Wally (Famous) Amos suggests that there might be something more than a homonymical relationship between "cookie" and "kooky." A talent agent at William Morris who signed Simon and Garfunkel and represented the Supremes and Dionne Warwick, Amos decided to get into the food business after a high-profile client, Hugh Masekela, dumped him as an agent and another client, an actor, fractured his leg just before shooting a movie that promised to launch his career. Amos set up his first cookie stand on Sunset Boulevard in 1975 with funding from Marvin Gaye, among others. Unable to dig up the hard facts of the chocolate-chip cookie's origins, an associate of Amos's dreamed up some information to print on his store's bags: the cookie was born "in a tiny farmhouse kitchen in Lowell, Massachusetts," on what "has come to be known as Brown Thursday." Amos, who dressed in a Panama hat and embroidered shirt and adopted the salutation "Have a very brown day," admits that he was a more successful pitchman than he was a businessman or pastry chef. He may have found his way to the cover of *Time* magazine, but between 1985 and 1989 ownership of Famous Amos changed hands four times, leaving Wally Amos with less and less of a stake in the company that he started. (Like Amos, Debbie Fields and David Liederman no longer own the businesses that bear their names, though all three remain active in the cookie business.)

Meanwhile, the chocolate-chip cookie, the tribble of American baked goods, kept reproducing itself in copious and unexpected ways. There came the Chipwich, the Taste of Nature Cookie Dough Bite, and the Pookie (a pie coated with chocolate-chip-cookie dough). Perhaps none of these variations was more culinarily or culturally significant than the début, in 1984, of Ben & Jerry's Chocolate Chip Cookie Dough ice cream at their Burlington, Vermont, store. The idea came from an anonymous note left by a customer and was soon in high demand in their neighboring outlets. It took Ben & Jerry's five years to find a way to mechanize the process of hand-mixing the frozen cookie dough with the ice cream, but it proved profitable. By 1991, Chocolate Chip Cookie Dough replaced Heath Bar Crunch as the company's bestselling product. Two decades later, it is still among Ben & Jerry's favorites.

Needless to say, reading about all of this got me hankering for some chocolate-chip cookies. My mother often made cookies from scratch during my childhood, especially around the Christmas season, but lately, like many Americans, I have come to rely on Pepperidge Farms and Costco to do my baking for me. Wyman's book sent me back into the kitchen, where I baked several batches of chocolate-chip cookies from scratch while writing this book. There's no doubt that time and a modicum of elbow grease are required to make cookies: it's harder than brewing a pot of coffee (unless you're Kelefa Sanneh) but easier, say, than making a bouillabaisse. For the most part, I stuck with the classic recipe printed on the back of the Nestlé package, but I benefited from having read David Leite's 2008 *NY Times* article on baking the perfect cookie. Leite advocated baking larger cookies than Wakefield's in order to produce a more appealing variety of textures. And while it kills spontaneity, his suggestion, gleaned from professional chefs, of letting the dough cool in a refrigerator for thirty-six hours before baking, is an invaluable one.

There are, of course, hundreds of other recipes I could have used. (Wyman prints some seventy-five in her thorough and entertaining book.) The beauty of the chocolate-chip cookie—and no small part of its enduring popularity—is its fungibility. You can make it with shortening, margarine, or butter; you can make big cookies or small cookies; you can use pecans or walnuts or M. & M.'s or peanut butter; you can use more brown sugar or less; you can swap in corn syrup or molasses; add an extra egg or substitute water for milk; you can use luxury brands of sea salt and caramel and extremely expensive hand-made chocolate or the generic brands available in your local supermarket. It doesn't matter. What comes out will still be recognizable as a chocolate-chip cookie and, most likely, it will taste good. It will go well with milk, sure, and coffee and tea, but I'm here to tell you that it will also taste great with red wine or whiskey. It seems that the only thing you can't do to a cookie, as Malcolm Gladwell discovered in

2005, is make it truly healthy. In its ability to absorb such a heterogeneous list of ingredients and still retain its identity and appeal, the chocolate-chip cookie is representative of the aspirations of the country for which it has become the preferred treat.

Eating my cookies, I thought about Ruth Wakefield's disinclination to discuss her most famous creation later in life. Nowadays, we'd expect the inventor of such an iconic bit of Americana to publish an autobiography and make regular appearances on the Food Network, but Wakefield didn't grandstand. A Toll House neighbor suggested to Wyman that Wakefield had "moved on," especially after she and her husband sold the restaurant, in 1967. (Wakefield died in 1977.) Wyman thinks it is possible that Wakefield, a successful businesswoman and cookbook author, didn't want her other achievements to be overshadowed by her celebrated cookie which, after all, had been invented merely as an accompaniment for ice cream. Wakefield's pecan rolls, Boston cream pie, and Indian pudding were enormously popular before being supplanted by the Toll House cookie. There are numerous other desserts from her "Tried and True" cookbook that are probably worth a second look, and during the holidays I aim to give a couple of them a shot.

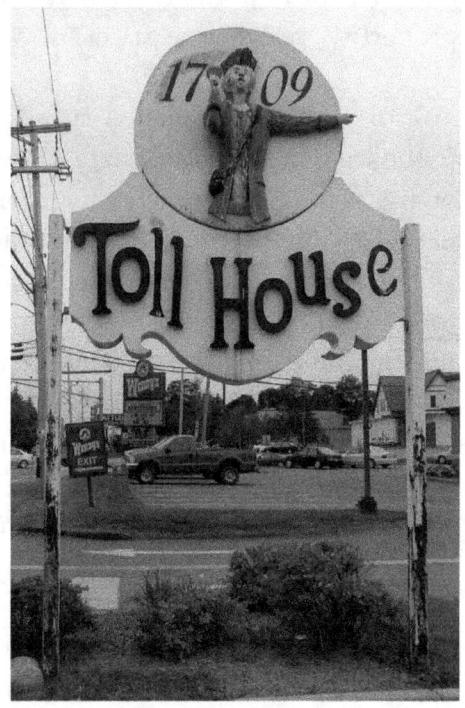

The Toll House restaurant burned down spectacularly on New Year's Eve in 1984 and the spot is now home to a Wendy's. The authorities in Whitman required that the fast-food restaurant include a small museum to Wakefield and the Toll House on its premises. Next time you're on the road between Boston and New Bedford, drop in and have a look. But, whatever you do, don't order a cookie. Instead, bake a batch from scratch when you get home!

4. Hershey's Chocolate

The rapid development of the chocolate-making industry in late 19th century did not escape the keen eye of one American confectioner; Milton Hershey. Building on the success of his Lancaster Caramel Company, Hershey began producing sweet chocolate and cocoa for flavoring and coating his own caramels in 1894. With the sale of his Lancaster Caramel Company to the American Caramel Company in August 1900 for $1,000,000 (over $27,000,000 in 2017 dollars,) Hershey now had the money to expand his chocolate business. After exploring several sites in and around Lancaster, Pennsylvania, Hershey decided to construct his new factory in a completely new location. After considering several urban sites along the eastern seaboard, Milton Hershey rejected traditional urban locations for his chocolate factory and instead decided to place his business in the country. He chose a site in Derry Township, near the place of his birth where he already owned property and could purchase additional property at reasonable prices.

Milton Hershey picked rural Derry Township against the advice of friends and business associates. They saw isolation. He saw a ready supply of fresh milk for his chocolate and a steady labor force made up of hardworking Pennsylvania Germans. His advisors saw the tiny town of Derry Church. Mr. Hershey envisioned a complete, new community. The town quickly emerged, following a plan that had been carefully thought out by Mr. Hershey. Workmen started digging the foundation for the Hershey chocolate factory in early 1903. Before the year was half over, a school and several other key buildings were also underway. In designing his community, Mr. Hershey was influenced by other "manufacturing communities" which were springing up at the turn of the century, both in this country and abroad.

Like other "model towns" Hershey provided its residents with a wholesome environment, modern educational facilities, and affordable housing. What set Hershey apart from similar towns, however, was that Mr. Hershey promoted it as a destination for tourists.

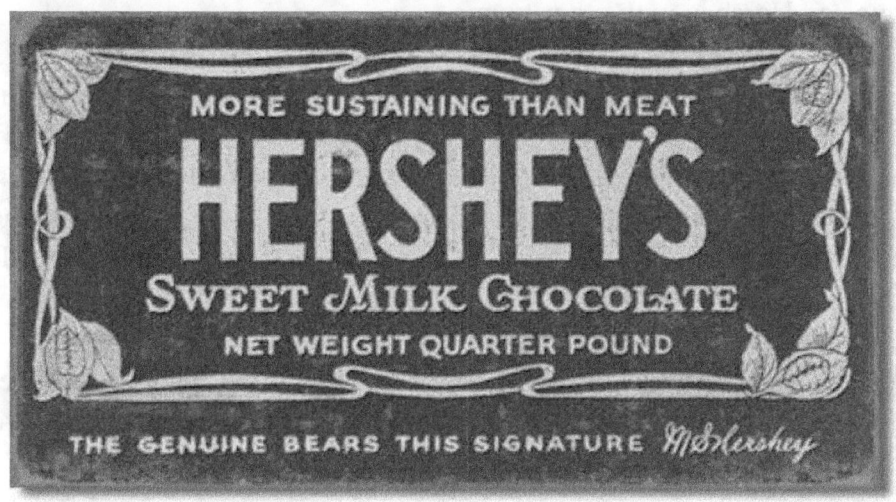

The first factory buildings were one story high and covered six acres. The original factory was designed and built to manufacture chocolate in the most efficient way possible. Raw materials, cocoa beans, milk, sugar, were delivered at one end of the factory and processed, emerging at the other end as finished products ready to be transported to market.

The key to the success of Hershey's chocolate was the mass production of a few high-quality items, including Hershey's milk chocolate and Hershey's breakfast cocoa in 1905; Hershey's Kisses chocolates in 1907; and Hershey's milk chocolate bar with almonds in 1908. Between 1910 and 1925, the ever-growing demand of consumers saw the factory increase its floor space from 18 acres in 1911 to 35 acres by 1915.

When Milton Hershey chose a rural site for his chocolate factory, he also envisioned building a completely new community. When the factory began to produce chocolate in June 1905, many buildings and public works considered to be essential by Milton Hershey were already in place. The most prominent of these buildings was the Cocoa House (which housed a bank, post office, general store, and several boarding rooms) as well as a consolidated public school called the McKinley School. Rail and trolley lines, laid out to transport workers and raw materials to the factory, also connected Hershey with other towns.

While ground was being broken for the new factory, newspapers and trade magazines published articles outlining Mr. Hershey's plans for his new factory and town. Hershey encouraged the curiosity and interest in his plans, knowing the benefits of effective publicity. Milton Hershey capitalized on the public's interest in his town from its inception. He included postcards of the town of Hershey in his nickel chocolate bars from 1909 until 1918. In 1915, Hershey opened a visitor's bureau and began to offer chocolate factory tours. By 1935, more than 50,000 people a year toured the factory. In 1916, the Hershey Zoo, the largest free private zoo in America at the time, opened to the public.

During the Great Depression of the 1930s, Milton Hershey took advantage of a ready and able supply of labor and cheap raw materials to embark on upon a massive building and public works projects to benefit his community and its growing number of visitors. Because of his vision, Milton Hershey constructed numerous facilities designed to meet a wide range of recreational, cultural, and educational needs which still benefit the community today. These buildings included: The Hershey Community Building, completed in 1932; the Hotel Hershey, completed in 1933; the Junior/Senior High School (now Catherine Hall) of the Hershey Industrial School (now Milton Hershey School), completed in 1934; the Windowless Office Building of the Hershey Chocolate Company (now the Hershey Company), completed in 1935; the Hershey Sports Arena, completed in 1936, and the Hershey Stadium, completed in 1939. Along with resources like Hershey Park, founded in 1907, Hershey Museum, founded in 1933, and Hershey Rose Garden, founded in 1936, Hershey emerged as a nationally known tourist destination by the end of the decade.

Though Milton Hershey passed away on October 13, 1945, the town and chocolate company as well as the various philanthropies and other industries which bear his name continue to keep his dream and vision alive.

During the Second World War, chocolate was an important part of the US war effort. Military chocolate has been a part of standard United States military ration since the original Ration D or D ration bar of 1937. Today, military chocolate is issued to troops as part of basic field rations and sundry packs. Chocolate rations served two purposes: as a morale boost, and as a high-energy, pocket-sized emergency ration. Military chocolate rations are often made in special lots to military specifications for weight, size, and endurance. The majority of chocolate issued to military personnel is produced by the Hershey Company.

When provided as a morale boost or care package, military chocolate is often no different from normal store-bought bars in taste and composition. However, they are frequently packaged or molded differently. The World War II K ration issued in temperate climates sometimes included a bar of Hershey's commercial-formula sweet chocolate. But instead of being the typical flat thin bar, the K ration chocolate was a thick rectangular bar that was square at each end (in tropical regions, the K ration used Hershey's Tropical Bar formula).

When provided as an emergency field ration, military chocolate was very different from normal bars. Since its intended use was as an emergency food source, it was formulated so that it would not be a tempting treat that troops might consume before they needed it. Even as attempts to improve the flavor were made, the heat-resistant chocolate bars never received rave reviews. Emergency ration chocolate bars were made to be high in energy value, easy to carry, and able to withstand high temperatures. Withstanding high temperatures was critical since infantrymen would often be outdoors, sometimes in tropical or desert conditions, with the bars located close to their bodies. These conditions would cause typical chocolate bars to melt within minutes.

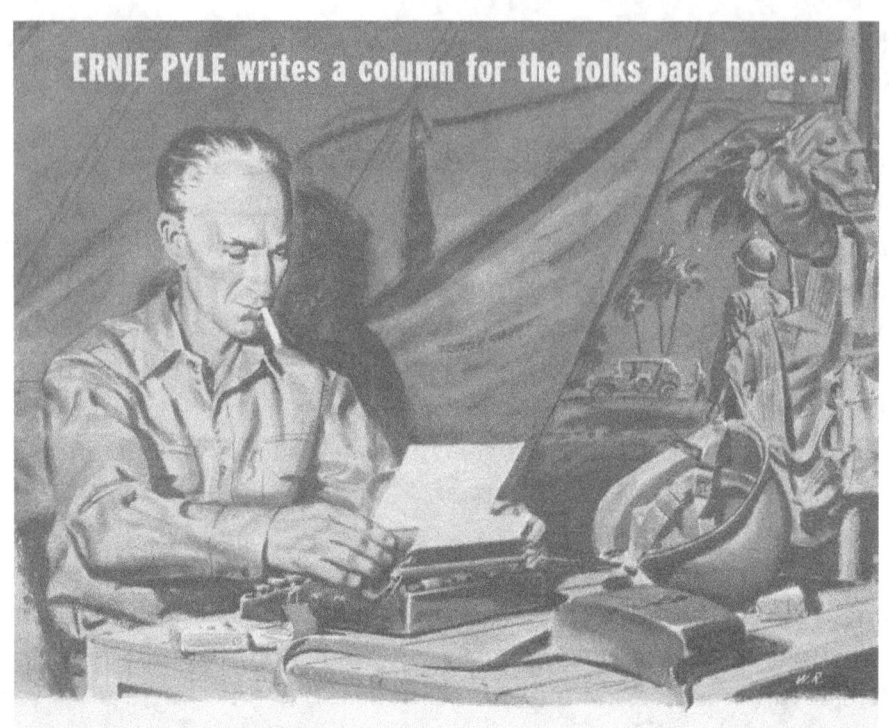

ERNIE PYLE writes a column for the folks back home...

"U.S. TROOPS FIGHT ON CHOCOLATE DIET"

The first emergency chocolate ration bar commissioned by the United States Army was the Ration D, commonly known as the D ration. Army Quartermaster Colonel Paul Logan approached Hershey's Chocolate in April 1937, and met with William Murrie, the company president, and Sam Hinkle, the chief chemist. Milton Hershey was extremely interested in the project when he was informed of the proposal, and the meeting began the first experimental production of the D ration bar.

Colonel Logan had four requirements for the D Ration Bar. The bar must:

1. Weigh 4 ounces (112 g)
2. Be high in food energy value
3. Be able to withstand high temperatures
4. Taste "a little better than a boiled potato"

Its ingredients were chocolate, sugar, oat flour, cacao fat, skim milk powder, and artificial flavoring. Chocolate manufacturing equipment was built to move the flowing mixture of liquid chocolate and oat flour into preset molds. However, the temperature-resistant formula of chocolate became a gooey paste that would not flow at any temperature.

Chief chemist Hinkle was forced to develop entirely new production methods to produce the bars. Each four-ounce portion had to be kneaded, weighed, and pressed into a mold by hand. The end result was an extremely hard block of dark brown chocolate that would crumble with some effort and was heat-resistant to 120 °F (49 °C). The resultant bar was wrapped in aluminum foil. Three bars sealed in a parchment packet made up a daily ration and was intended to furnish the individual combat soldier with the 1,800 calories (7,500 kJ) minimum sustenance recommended each day.

Colonel Logan was pleased with the first small batch of samples. In June 1937, the United States Army ordered 90,000 D ration or "Logan Bars" and field tested them at bases in the Philippines, Panama, on the Texas border, and at other bases throughout the United States. Some of the bars even found their way into the supplies for Admiral Byrd's third Antarctic expedition. These field tests were successful, and the Army began making regular orders for the bars. With the onset of America's involvement in World War II after the attack on Pearl Harbor, the bars were ordered to be packaged to make them poison gas proof. The 4-ounce (112 g) bars' boxes were covered with an anti-gas coating and were packed 12 to a cardboard carton, which was also coated.

These cartons were packed 12 to a wooden crate for a total of 144 bars to a crate. Colonel Logan had specified that the D ration taste only a bit better than "a boiled potato." This last requirement was imposed to keep soldiers from eating their emergency rations in non-emergency situations. As a result, the D ration was almost universally detested for its bitter taste by U.S. troops, and was often discarded instead of consumed when issued. Troops called the D ration "Hitler's Secret Weapon" for its effect on soldiers' intestinal tracts. It could not be eaten at all by soldiers with bad or even false teeth, and even those with good dental work often found it necessary to first shave slices off the bar with a knife before consuming.

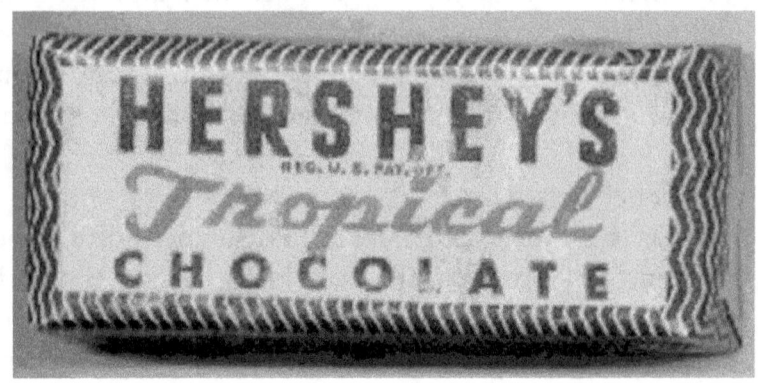

In 1943, the Procurement Division of the Army approached Hershey about producing a confectionery-style chocolate bar with improved flavor that would still withstand extreme heat for issue in the Pacific Theater. After a short period of experimentation, the Hershey company began producing Hershey's Tropical Bar. The bar was designed for issue with field and specialty rations, such as the K ration, and originally came in 1-ounce (28 g) and 2-ounce (56 g) sizes. After 1945, it came in 4-ounce (112 g) D ration sizes as well.

The Tropical Bar (it was called the D ration throughout the war, despite its new appellation) had more of a resemblance to normal chocolate bars in its shape and flavor than the original D ration, which it gradually replaced by 1945. While attempts to sweeten its flavor were somewhat successful, nearly all U.S. soldiers found the Tropical Bar tough to chew and unappetizing; reports from countless memoirs and field reports are almost uniformly negative. Instead, the bar was either discarded or traded to unsuspecting Allied troops or civilians for more appetizing foods or goods.

Resistance to accepting the ration soon appeared among the latter groups after the first few trades. In the Burma theater of war (CBI), the D ration or Tropical Bar did make one group of converts: it was known as the "dysentery ration", since the bar was the only ration those ill with dysentery could tolerate.

In 1957, the bar's formula was changed to make it more appetizing. The unpopular oat flour was removed, 'non-fat milk solids' replaced 'skim-milk powder', 'Cocoa powder' replaced 'cacao fat', and artificial vanilla flavoring was added. It was added with the help of sugar. It greatly improved the flavor of the bar, but it was still difficult to chew. During the war years, the "bulk of the Hershey Food Corporation's chocolate production was for the military. Between 1940 and 1945, an estimated 3 billion units of the specially formulated candy bars were distributed to soldiers around the world." This chocolate ration was part of a larger scale of rationed foodstuffs. The ideology of food, as seen by U.S. propaganda director Elmer Davis is suggested to be "a profoundly political matter during the Second World War. As global famine conditions and national rationing programs came to define the daily lives of most people, agriculture and eating became fraught emblems of military power, war trade, and political allegiances."

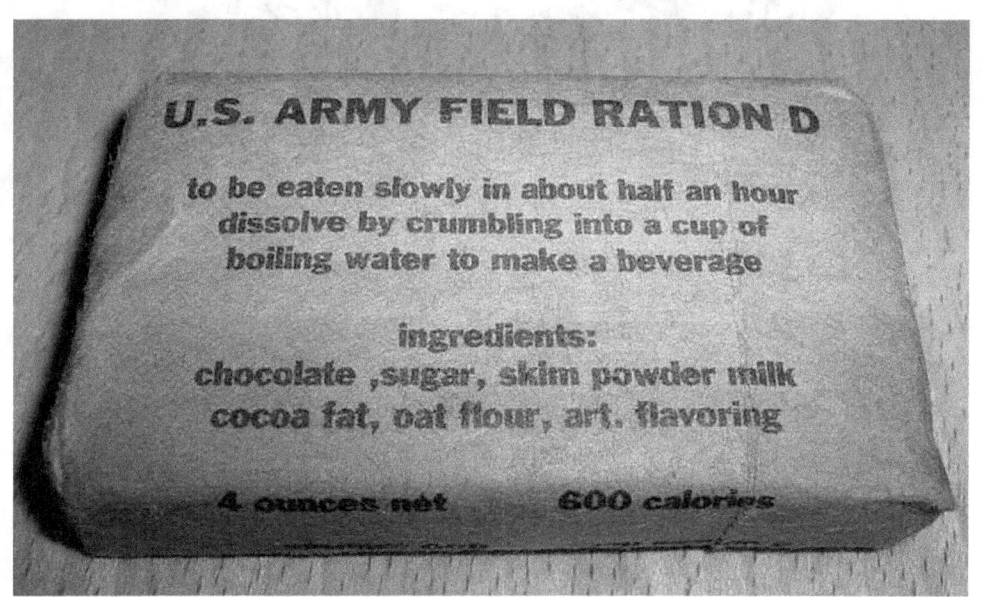

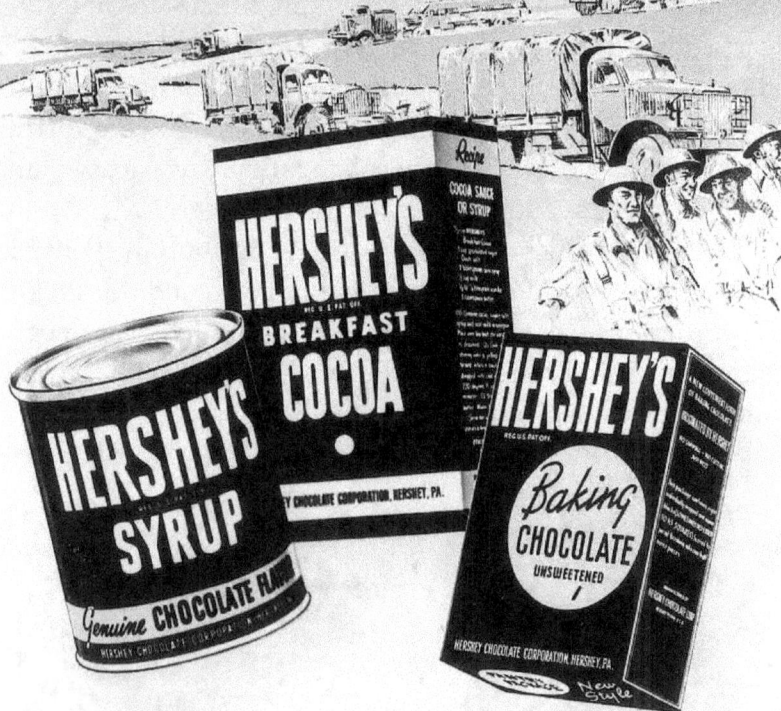

Supplying—
OUR ARMED FORCES

LIMITS THE QUANTITY *for you...*

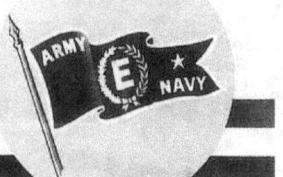

Buy War Bonds and Stamps

It is estimated that between 1940 and 1945, over 3 billion of the D ration and Tropical Bars were produced and distributed to soldiers throughout the world. In 1939, the Hershey plant was capable of producing 100,000 ration bars a day. By the end of World War II, the entire Hershey plant was producing ration bars at a rate of 24 million a week. For their service throughout World War II, the Hershey Chocolate Company was issued the Army-Navy 'E' Award for Excellence for exceeding expectations for quality and quantity in the production of the D ration and the Tropical Bar. Their continued efforts resulted in four stars being added to their pennant signifying the five times they received this distinction. U.S. propaganda used this product distinction during the war as a message "that Allied nations would win the war because of their democratic institutions, but also because of the productivity of the U.S. economy and, especially, its agriculture."

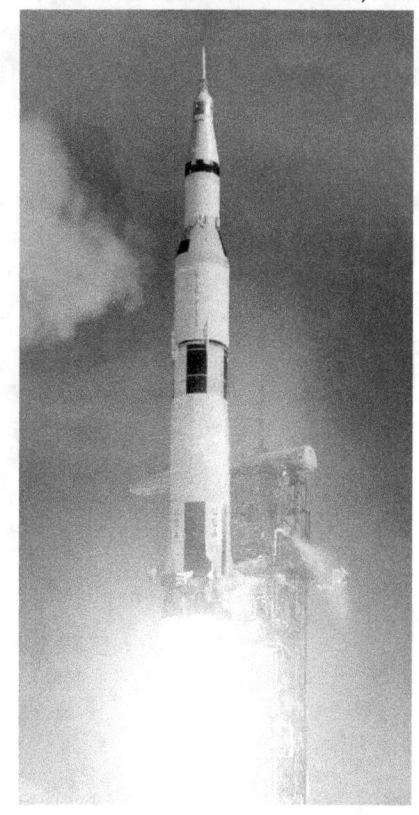

Production of the D ration bar was discontinued at the end of World War II. However, Hershey's Tropical Bar remained a standard ration for the United States Armed Forces. The Tropical Bar saw action in Korea and Vietnam as an element of the "Sundries" kit (which also contained toiletries), before being declared obsolete.

In July of 1971, chocolate even accompanied the crew of Apollo 15 on their journey to the moon. Proving for all time that **chocolate is indeed out of the world!**

5. Wine in History

According to an ancient Persian fable, wine was the accidental discovery of a princess seeking to end her life with what she thought was poison. Instead, she found wine and it has been welcome part of our culture ever since! Evolving over the centuries, grape growing and wine-making has continued to grip the human imagination, inspiring passion and ingenuity.

Archeological evidence suggests that grape cultivation and wine making began in Mesopotamia and areas surrounding the Caspian Sea sometime between 6000 and 4000 BC. The drink was savored by royalty

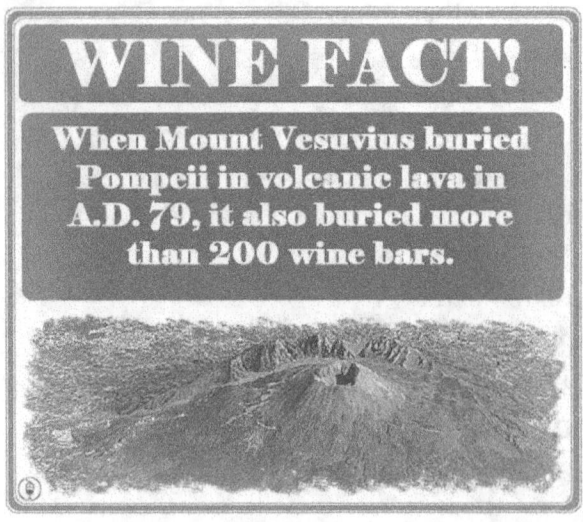

WINE FACT!

When Mount Vesuvius buried Pompeii in volcanic lava in A.D. 79, it also buried more than 200 wine bars.

and priests, while commoners drank beer, mead, and ale. The ancient Egyptians, the first culture known to document the process of wine making, preserved descriptions of harvesting grapes and drinking wine on clay tablets, which have been discovered within the burial chambers of the social elite.

Wine making made its way to Greece, where it permeated all aspects of society: literature, mythology, medicine, leisure, and religion. The Romans took vine clippings from Greece back to Italy, and centers of viticulture soon developed in France, Germany, Italy, Spain, Portugal, and the rest of Europe.

Trade routes and early explorers carried vines and grape growing treatises to Mexico, Argentina, and North Africa, and the culture of wine continues to spread around the globe today, with vines growing on every continent except Antarctica.

Wine has been a popular beverage of mankind for thousands of years. Our natural fondness of this drink stems from the wonderful taste, its nutritious properties and not least its psychotropic (intoxicating) effects.

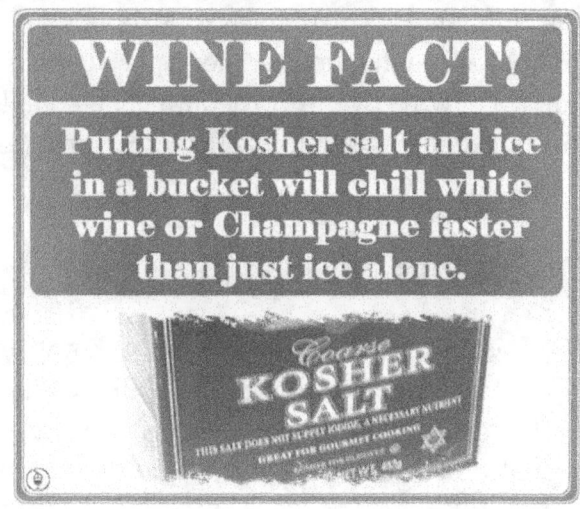

WINE FACT!

Putting Kosher salt and ice in a bucket will chill white wine or Champagne faster than just ice alone.

Out of all alcoholic drinks, none has had such an impact on society. The trade of wine between cultures opened up channels for religious and philosophical ideas to spread across Europe. Wine is also frequently mentioned in the bible from Noah and his grape vines to Jesus, as perhaps the finest winemaker to date.

Wine is to this day used in the Catholic Church as a substitute for the blood of Christ, which is an indication of the key role the beverage has played in years gone by. Centuries ago, a wine industry was also the mark of a provident country, as only developed societies could support a prosperous and competitive wine industry. It is often said that western society built its foundations on wine.

One path of wine history could follow the developments and science of grape growing and wine production; another might separately trace the spread of wine commerce through civilization, but there would be many crossovers and detours between them. No matter how one chooses to follow the time line, it is clear that wine and human history have greatly influenced one another.

Fossil vines, 60-million-years-old, are the earliest scientific evidence of grapes. The earliest written account of viniculture is in the Old Testament of the Bible which tells us that Noah planted a vineyard and made wine. As cultivated fermentable crops, honey and grain are older than grapes, many believe that neither mead nor beer has had anywhere near the social impact of wine over recorded time. Personally, I would argue that beer has had an equally great impact on our world (especially in Germany).

Ancient Wine History

The first sign of the wine we all know and love can be traced back to sixty-million-year-old fossils, which means our pre-human ancestors may well have come to realize older grapes will have been more desirable. We can also observe this with our animal friends today, who tend to prefer riper fruit.

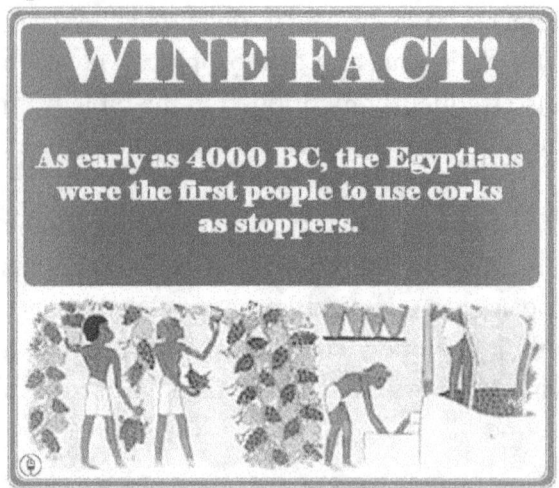

The earliest remnants of wine were discovered in the site of Hajji Firuz Tepe, in the northern Zagros Mountains of Iran. The wine dated back to the Neolithic period (8500-4000 BC). Carbon dating confirmed the wine was from sometime between 5400-5000 BC. Although wine dating any earlier than this has yet been found, it is thought the art of wine making started shortly after 6000 B.C. it is believed this is the date for one of mankind's most momentous creations, because the people of these regions had managed to create permanent settlements via the domestication of animals and plants.

This was a far more stable living situation than the Nomadic way of living, which most humans were currently employing. This stability allowed people to experiment with their cuisine and drinks. Some of our favorite dishes and drinks we still enjoy today were developed in this time period, including beer and, of course, wine.

Now we skip forward a few thousand years to the Predynastic era of the Egyptian Pharaohs, when wine was spreading across the ancient world. Hieroglyphics from this time show that perhaps binge drinking is not such a modern problem, as apparently, the Pharaohs didn't seem to care that much about the quality - but more on quantity.

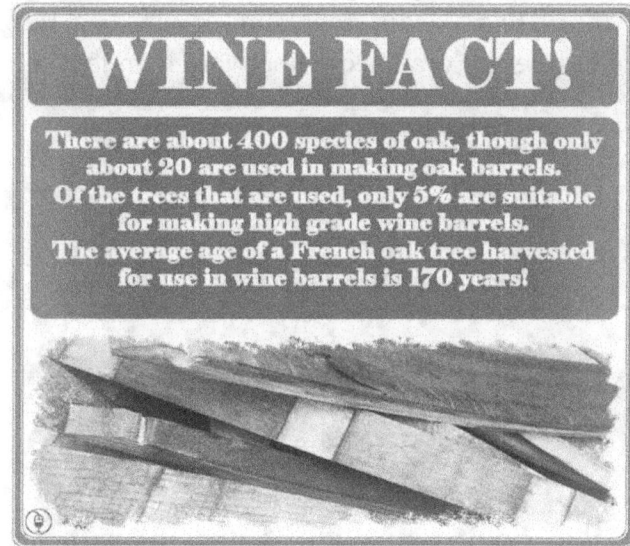

WINE FACT!

There are about 400 species of oak, though only about 20 are used in making oak barrels. Of the trees that are used, only 5% are suitable for making high grade wine barrels. The average age of a French oak tree harvested for use in wine barrels is 170 years!

However, the wine the Egyptians drank was a distant relative to the wine we know today. The Egyptians used white, pink, green, red, and dark blue grapes, as well as figs, palm, dates and pomegranates. So, as you can imagine, the taste would have been completely different to what we would expect when being served wine today. Making wine from various fruits is essentially the same as that of grapes, except sugar is added to help the fermentation.

The Egyptians used trellises, which were protected from sunlight (because the light is too intense in Egypt) and they also knew that the last 100 days before the harvest were the most vital. Once the grapes were picked they were taken to a large pressing vat. The Egyptians pressed grapes by treading on them, rather than using a stone press to crush the seeds and stems, adding a bitter taste to the resulting wine.

There was then a second pressing of the wine in an oblong linen slough. This slough was stretched across a solid wooden frame as four men on one side stretched the linen, meanwhile a fifth made sure none of the precious wine was spilt.

The Egyptians had several grades of wine:

- Free Run Must: Little of this was collected, but it was a very sweet long lasting wine
- First Wine Must: This came from the treading and was about 2/3 of the juice
- Second Run Must: This came from the additional pressing.

These 3 grades could be mixed to make different kinds of wine (e.g. red, white, dry or sweet). These 3 different grades of wine were then left in a trough to ferment.

It seems that the Pharaohs were particularly fond of the drink, as it became their preference to take into the afterlife. At this time, wine was almost exclusively for royalty and served only at special occasions like festivals. However, it also had medical uses like sedating women during childbirth and as an antiseptic.

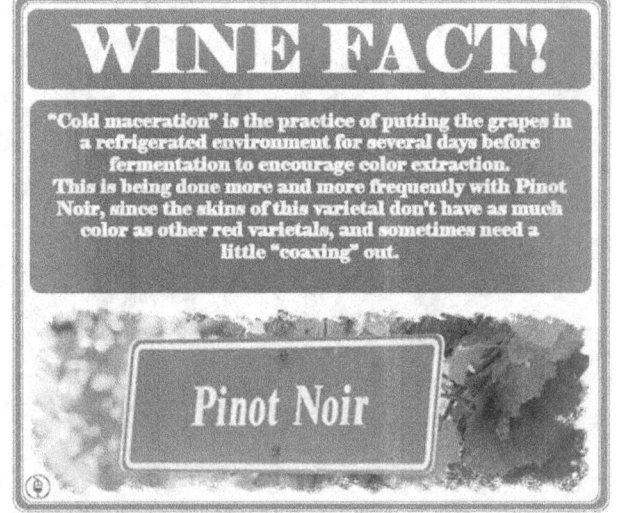

WINE FACT!

"Cold maceration" is the practice of putting the grapes in a refrigerated environment for several days before fermentation to encourage color extraction. This is being done more and more frequently with Pinot Noir, since the skins of this varietal don't have as much color as other red varietals, and sometimes need a little "coaxing" out.

Pinot Noir

When sealing their wine, Egyptians would make an impression in the wax. These were the equivalent to the wine maker's labels we have today.

We know that wine has been around and has been enjoyed for eons. Over 4000 years ago, during the rule of The Third Dynasty of Ur, also known as the Neo-Sumerian Empire, we know that they enjoyed wine. We

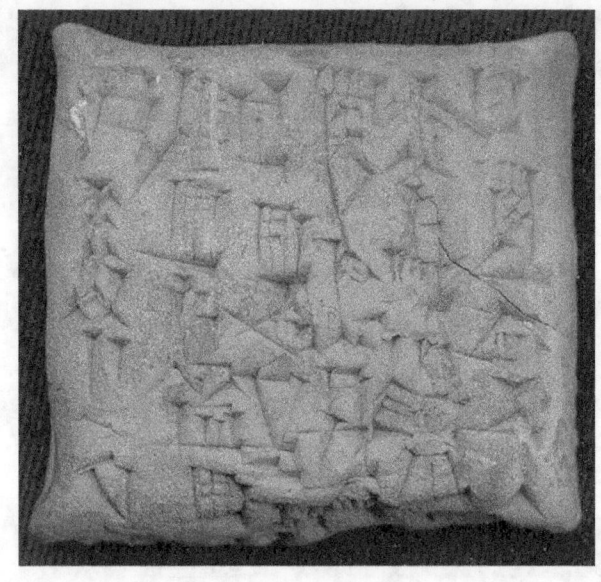

know because we have found an ancient clay Cuneiform tablet, dating from 2031 BC.

This small, clay tablet dates from the sixth year of Shu-Sin (2031 BCE), fourth king of the Third Dynasty of Ur (2112-2004 BCE). The tablet records perhaps the earliest documented mention of wine. It is a receipt for jugs of wine from the supervisor of the estate as received by the estate cook, Adalal.

Cuneiform, from the Latin *cuneus*, meaning "wedge," is the term applied to a mode of writing which used a wedge-shaped stylus to make impressions on a clay surface, or on stone, metal, or wax. Most clay tablets were baked in the heat of the desert sun, it is truly amazing that something this old and fragile has survived long enough to be discovered and treasured by modern archeologists.

We know that wine was enjoyed during biblical times though some suggest that the "wine" they enjoyed was actually nonalcoholic grape juice. It is often supposed that in Bible times, grape juice inevitably fermented if kept for any length of time and that therefore whenever the Bible mentions "wine," it is referring to the alcoholic beverage commonly called "wine" today. However, ancient civilizations had several ways of preventing fruit and fruit juices from fermentation, and thus were able to have non-alcoholic wine (grape juice) throughout the year.

One method involved boiling the juice and reducing it to a syrup that could later be diluted with water. Another was to boil the juice with minimum evaporation and then immediately seal it with beeswax in airtight jars. Drying the fruit in the sun and then reconstituting it with water, adding sulfur to the fruit juice, or filtering the juice to extract the gluten were also methods that would prevent the juice from fermenting. These means of preservation were known to the ancients, who also practiced boiling fermented juice to eliminate the alcohol. Referring to reconstituting grape syrup to make grape juice, Aristotle, who was born around 384 BC, wrote "The wine of Arcadia was so thick that it was necessary to scrape it from the skin bottles in which it was contained and to dissolve the scrapings in water" (quoted in Nott's Lectures on Biblical Temperance, p. 80). The poet Horace, born in 65 BC wrote, "There is no wine sweeter to drink than that of Lesbos; it was like nectar . . . and would not produce intoxication."

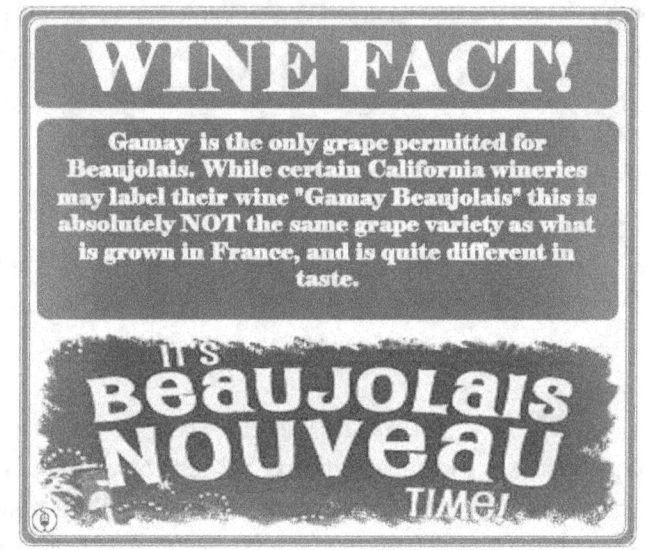

"The Mishna [a collection of oral Jewish traditions] states that the Jews were in the habit of drinking boiled wine" (Kitto's Cyclopedia of Biblical Literature, vol. 2, p. 447). Naturally, this wine would be entirely free of alcohol as a result of the boiling, if not also from the manner of preservation.

In his commentary on the Gospel of John, Albert Barnes wrote, "The wine of Judea was the pure juice of the grape, without any mixture of alcohol. It was the common drink of the people and did not produce intoxication." And Adam Clarke, commenting on Genesis 40:11, wrote, "From this we find that wine anciently was the mere expressed juice of the grape without fermentation. The saky, or cupbearer, took the bunch [of grapes], pressed the juice into the cup, and instantly delivered it into the hands of his master. This was anciently the yayin [wine] of the Hebrews, the oinos [wine] of the Greeks, and the mustum [wine] of the ancient Latins."

But then others point out that in the very first book of the Bible, Genesis, mentions a wine that was indeed alcohol. Genesis 20 and 21 state:

*"After the flood, Noah began to cultivate the ground, and he planted a vineyard. One day he drank some wine he had made, **and he became drunk** and lay naked inside his tent."*

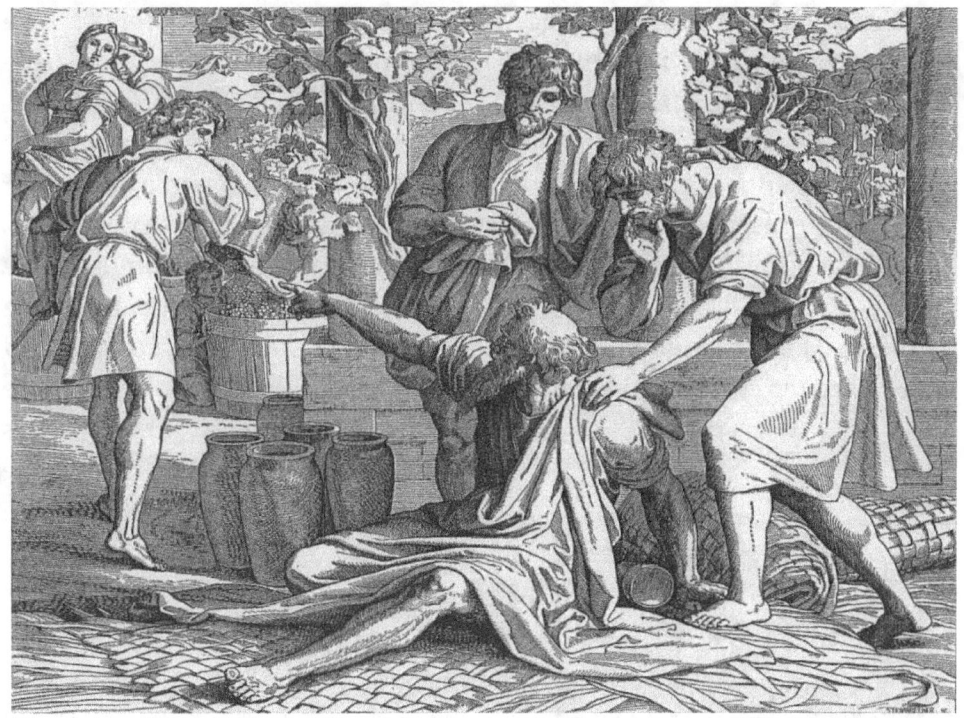

Look, I honestly think that it really doesn't matter whether the wine during biblical times was free of alcohol or not. Either way, it was still wine and it was still enjoyed!

The ancient Persian fable mentioned above credits a lady of the court with the discovery of wine. This Princess, having lost favor with her father, the King, attempted to poison herself by eating some table grapes that had "spoiled" in a jar. She became intoxicated and giddy and fell asleep. When she awoke, she found the stresses that had made her life intolerable had dispersed. Returning to the source of her relief, she ate again of the "spoiled" grapes, her subsequent conduct changed so remarkably that she regained the King's favor. He shared his daughter's discovery with his court and decreed that there must be an increase in the production of "spoiled" grapes...

Although this is a pleasant tale, the accidental discovery of wine probably happened a few times in different regions, but what is sure is that the invention of wine must go down to pure dumb luck. Certainly wine, as a natural phase of grape spoilage, was "discovered" by accident, unlike beer and bread, which are human inventions. It is established that wine drinking had started by about 4000 BC and possibly as early as 6000 BC. The first efforts at grape cultivation can be traced to the area that forms the "Fertile Crescent", around the Caspian Sea and in Mesopotamia, including portions of present-day Georgia, Armenia, Azerbaijan, Iran, and Turkey. Excavations from tombs in ancient Egypt prove that wine was in use there by 3100 BC. Priests and royalty enjoyed wine, while beer was drunk by the workers. The Egyptians recognized differences in wine quality and developed the first arbors and pruning methods. Archeologists have uncovered many sites with sunken jars, so the effects of temperature on stored wine were probably known.

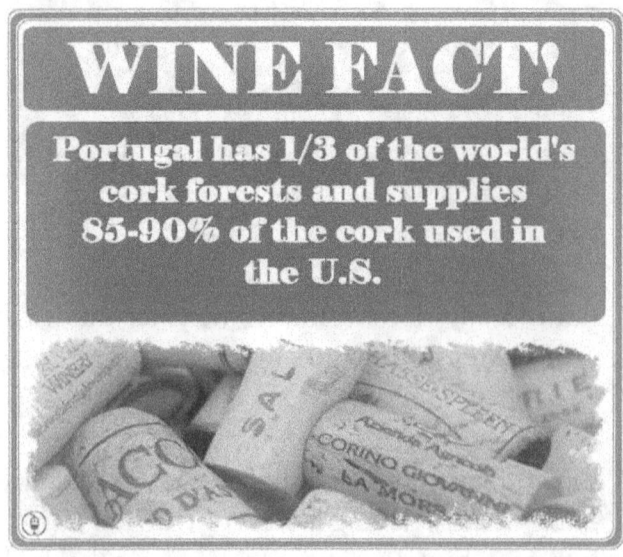

WINE FACT!

Portugal has 1/3 of the world's cork forests and supplies 85-90% of the cork used in the U.S.

Wine came to Europe with the spread of the Greek civilization around 1600 BC. Homer's *Odyssey* and *Iliad* both contain excellent and detailed descriptions of wine.

Wine was an important article of Greek commerce and Greek doctors, including Hippocrates, were among the first to prescribe it. The Greeks also learned to add herbs and spices to mask spoilage. The early signs of the wine in Greece were the replica wine presses found in Crete tombs and date back to between 3000BC-2000BC.

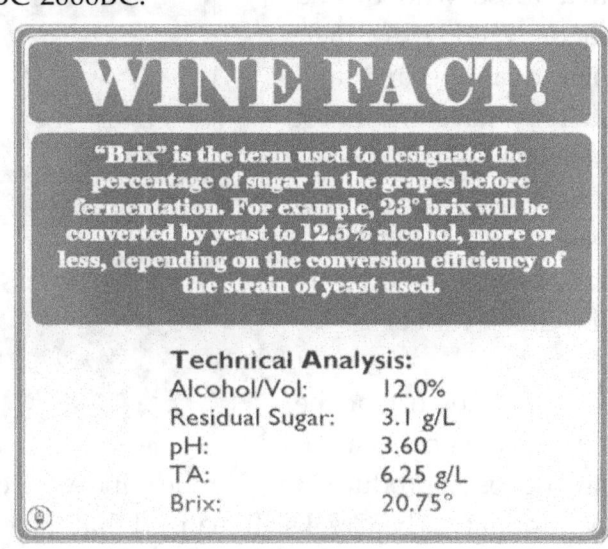

It is believed the Phoenician traders introduced the Greeks to the joys of wine. After the Phoenicians did the Greeks this favor, wine industries were established in most of Western Europe. Alexander the Great also introduced the drink to Asia.

WINE FACT!

"Brix" is the term used to designate the percentage of sugar in the grapes before fermentation. For example, 23° brix will be converted by yeast to 12.5% alcohol, more or less, depending on the conversion efficiency of the strain of yeast used.

Technical Analysis:

Alcohol/Vol:	12.0%
Residual Sugar:	3.1 g/L
pH:	3.60
TA:	6.25 g/L
Brix:	20.75°

The Greeks knew the nutritional benefits of drinking wine, which is an excuse we still all use today! In ancient Greece, the wine was so important it developed a religious status. They valued wine highly and referred to it as "The juice of the Gods." It couldn't have described better. There's also the Greek God of wine, Dionysus, who's the son of Zeus and one of the most worshiped Gods.

The Greeks used wine to achieve clarity of mind when at a symposia (a gathering where predetermined philosophical subjects were discussed). They would never drink wine as some people today do and drunkenness was frowned upon. This is a great indication of how thoroughly embedded in the culture wine traditions were.

By looking at the countries the Greeks introduced winemaking to, we can get a vague idea of how the ancient Greeks made wine and how it may have tasted. Another clue to the flavor of the wine is the surviving Greek varieties such as Limnio, Athiri, Aidani and Muscat.

The ancient Greek wine became so popular in Europe that vine cuttings from Greece's grapes became very prized so that those who owned them could grow their own quality grapes and thereby have the finest of wine. This, of course, means that many of the grape varieties we know today were fathered by the Greek varieties.

WINE FACT!

Tears (sometimes referred to as "legs") develop and flow down the sides of glass following swirling. They are little more than a basic indicator of the wine's alcohol content. The thicker and more prominant the legs, the higher the percentage of alcohol.

It is known that the regions of Hios, Thassos and Levos all produced high-grade wine, whereas the wines of Samos were poor quality. The Greeks all realized that the ecosystem played a key role in the characteristics of the resulting wine. They were the first to create their own appellations of origin, anyone caught violating them received a severe penalty.

The ancient Greeks highly valued sweet wine, as they do today. This may have been due to its staying power, but more likely its popularity stemmed from the sweetness and higher alcohol percentage. It is no well-kept secret that the Greeks like to mix their wine with water (including sea water amazingly) and to add honey and spices. This, again, shows us of how thoroughly embedded in the culture wine traditions were.

During the Turkish occupation of Greece, their wine industry was almost whipped out as the Muslim Turks discouraged winemaking and heavily taxed wine farmers. This meant many farmers went out of business and the only people who were excluded from the heavy tax where monks.

Fortunately, the monasteries kept the craft alive in Greece for the 400 years it was occupied. The Greeks then achieved independence in 1821. The Greek farmers started to replace their vines with raisin producing vines, as there was a huge demand for them from France, who's vines had been devastated by the Phylloxera insect.

After France recovered, the demand for raisins went down and the Greeks started to grow wine vines again. Unfortunately, there were then a series of wars (WWI, WWII and the Greek Civil War). These prevented a stable wine trade from being established until 1949.

At first the winemakers just churned out standard table wine and it looked like the nation who first produced fine wines would never return to its former glory. Fortunately, though, the Greek winemakers are on the upswing and with an arsenal of 300 different native grape varieties - each with very distinctive flavors - they would soon resume their position as one of the leading producers and worldwide distributors of quality wine.

The next group to start developing winemaking and the actual growth of the vine in roughly 1000BC were, in fact, a Greek colony that had grown so strong they had become independent of the Greeks.

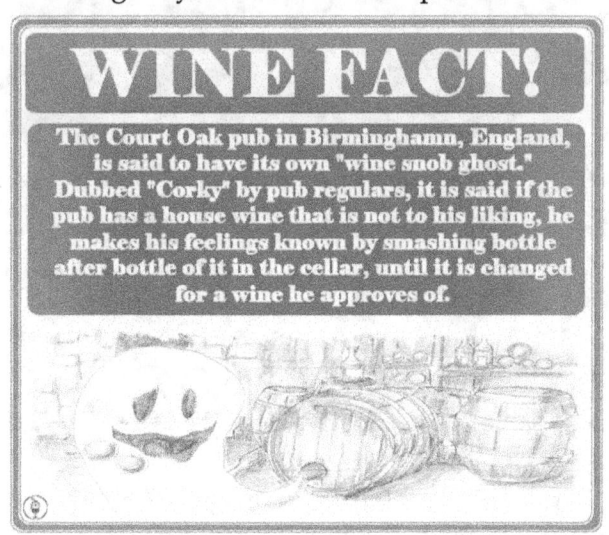

WINE FACT!

The Court Oak pub in Birminghamn, England, is said to have its own "wine snob ghost." Dubbed "Corky" by pub regulars, it is said if the pub has a house wine that is not to his liking, he makes his feelings known by smashing bottle after bottle of it in the cellar, until it is changed for a wine he approves of.

If you haven't guessed it yet, I am of course referring to the Romans. The Romans made major contributions to the science of winemaking. They took huge steps to the classification of many varieties of grapes. They also invented the wooden wine barrel. This was a huge development considering the kind of wood used to make the barrel imparts its own distinct flavors to the wine. Also, the barrels allow for the wine to evaporate a little bit during the aging process.

It is important to remember the Romans laid down the foundations of modern wine making. The Romans are also thought to be the first to use glass bottles for wine. The oldest bottle of wine to be found has been dated to 325 AD. Corking had been invented at that time, but the Romans preferred to preserve their wine by floating a layer of olive oil on it. They classified many diseases that afflict grapes.

At first the Romans didn't take to wine and sent any that was produced over the Alps to the barbarian Gauls, (modern day France) who were fond of the drink. The Romans preferred drink was beer and mead, because of their warrior past. Wine didn't really take off until the sacking of Carthage in 146 BC, because with the sacking they also acquired the first ever book about wine making.

Then Cato, (who suspiciously had pushed for the attack on Carthage) wrote a book on winemaking (which made him a fortune), called 'De Agi Cultura'. Thanks to this book, beer and mead were a thing of the past and wine was the drink of the future.

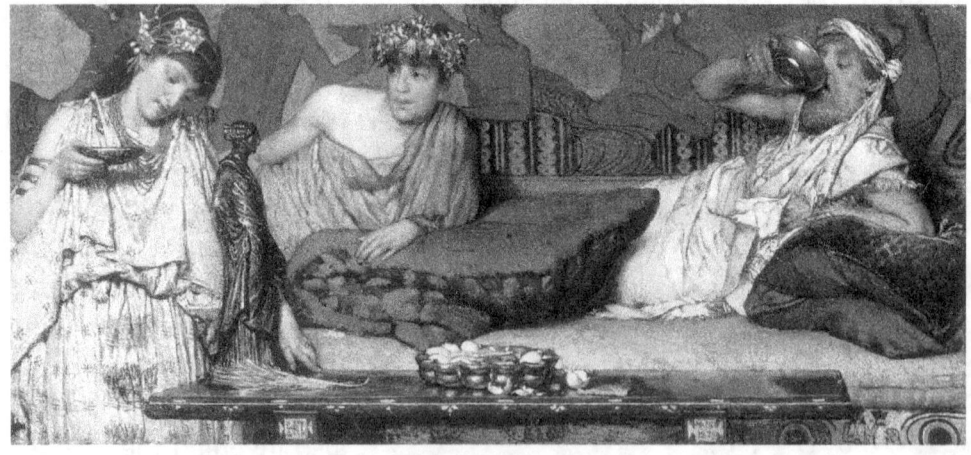

After another hundred years, there would be defined regions for winemaking. Apparently, the most desired regions were Falernian and Caecuban, but they disappeared after just 50 years due to Neronian public works. If the wine was as fine as it is claimed, then this conclusively proves the mental condition of Emperor Nero was very poor indeed.

The Romans, much like the Greeks, enjoyed drinking parties where philosophical debates and poetry readings took place. The difference in these parties was that the Romans tended to get very drunk and dancing girls and orgies were also a standard part of the night. The master of ceremonies would choose the type or blend of wine, how much water should be mixed with the wine 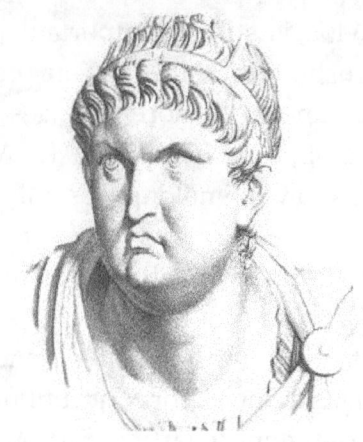 and call out the toasts. In short, he had the best job going at the party. The people who attended these parties were rich, but the poor got their fair share of wine also. At the theatre and at the games, there was a drink called muslum, which consisted of cheap wine mixed with honey. This was provided by politicians that needed support for the next election.

Wine wasn't just for merriment, it also had an important role in religion. It was consumed a lot at the graveside funeral feasts. Wine was poured down specially designed orifices in the tombs, so that the dead could share wine with the living. Wine continued to play a significant role in the Catholic religion.

No one can actually say what the Roman wine tasted like, but as with the Greeks, we can get a pretty good idea by the taste of wine made from the surviving varieties of grapes. Personally, I'd rather leave the mystery of the flavor of Roman wine as just that; a mystery. The other great contribution that Romans gave to winemaking was that every province they conquered, so we are talking about most of Western Europe, they established a wine industry. As the empire grew the wine in their province started to rival the wines being made in Rome, especially Portugal which became famous for its wine. The Romans therefore gave it the honor of naming it Lusitania, after their God of wine Lyssa (Bacchus). The amount of wine being produced was so great that in 92 AD Emperor Domitian decreed that half of the grape vines outside of Rome were to be uprooted.

Wine is still an important part of Italian culture and is taken very seriously, which this Italian proverb shows quite nicely: "One barrel of wine can work more miracles than a church full of saints." When the Roman Empire fell in 476 AD, Western Europe was plunged into the Dark Ages and winemaking was only kept alive by the Roman Catholic Church.

So even with all of the problems and horrors the Roman Empire wrought, the foundation and strength of viniculture in Western Europe must be primarily credited, to their influence. Starting about 1000 BC, the Romans made major contributions in classifying grape varieties and colors, observing and charting ripening characteristics, identifying diseases and recognizing soil-type preferences. They became skilled at pruning and increasing yields through irrigation and fertilization techniques. It was the Romans who were said to make the most delicious wine in ancient times.

The Romans also adapted wooden cooperage, an invention they acquired with the spoils of conquering Germanic tribes, to wine storage and transportation. This was a great advance for operations previously accomplished in skins or clay jars (amphora). They may also have been the first to use glass bottles, as glassblowing became more common during this era. Beginning about 200 BC, Roman exploits were as significant as Roman experiments as the armies of Rome planted wine vines in the wake of their conquests, all over the land mass now known as Europe.

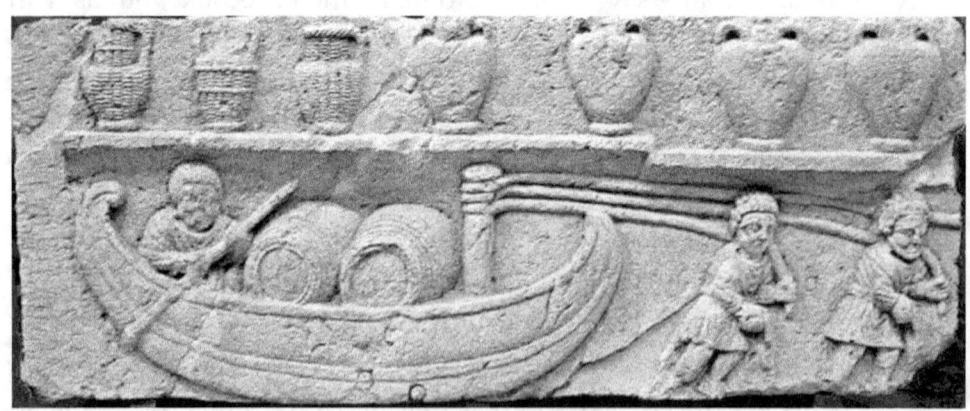

Modern Wine History

Monks of the Catholic Church, (particularly Benedictine monks) spread the knowledge of wine even further, as wine was required for Holy Communion. The Church transported it all across Europe, spreading the "good news" as it were. The only problem was, the wine they distributed was heavily watered down, as the Church didn't take kindly to drunkenness. Eventually, the French aristocracy took on the task of winemaking alongside the church.

Now let's take a quick moment to look at one of wine's proudest moments in its long history. I of course am referring to the creation of champagne. Despite common belief, champagne was not created by the monk, Dom Perignon, but was in fact researched 30 years earlier.

An English scientist and physician named Christopher Merrett presented findings to the Royal Society in 1662 called 'Some observations concerning the Ordering of wine.'

Champagne was reserved for very special occasions, such as French Coronation Festivities. Kings appreciated it so much they even sent it as homage to other monarchs. The reason for champagne being held with such high regard was that the pressure on the bottles often caused them to explode. Also, the explosion from one bottle disintegrating would often cause a chain reaction amongst other bottles. This meant that it was common to lose 20-90% of champagne. The bottles were so volatile that the monks brewing them had to wear heavy iron masks to protect themselves when in the cellars. The monks referred to champagne as "Devil's wine" and so strongly did they dislike it that Dom Perignon was sent down to the cellars with the specific job of getting rid of his Devil's wine.

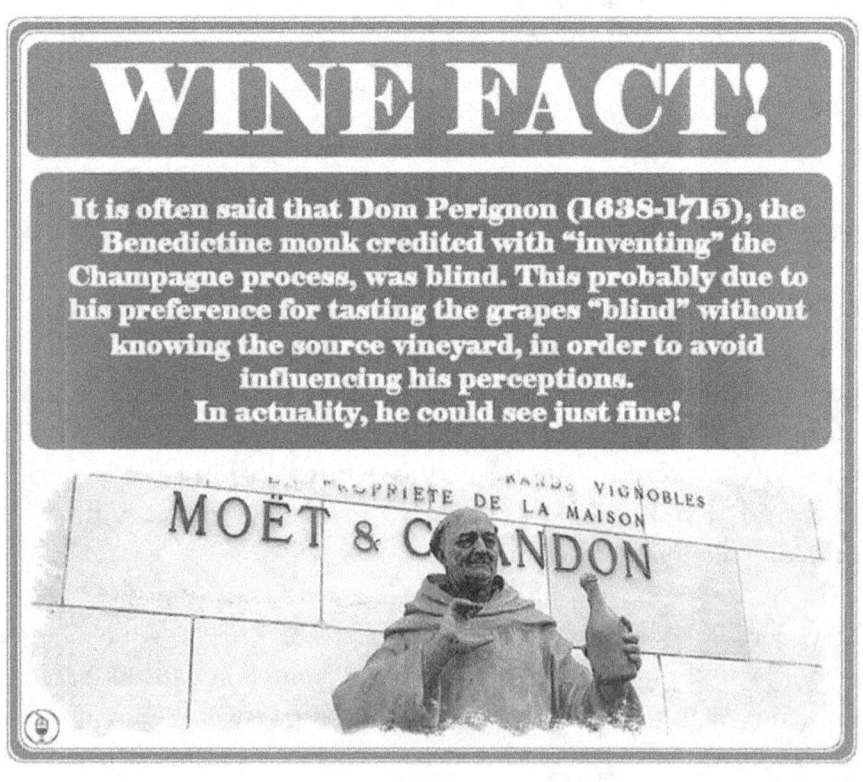

WINE FACT!

It is often said that Dom Perignon (1638-1715), the Benedictine monk credited with "inventing" the Champagne process, was blind. This probably due to his preference for tasting the grapes "blind" without knowing the source vineyard, in order to avoid influencing his perceptions.
In actuality, he could see just fine!

Fortunately for us all, Dom Perignon, was fond of the Devil's wine and instead invented techniques to accommodate the new sparkling. One was to thicken the glass of the wine bottles so they could withstand the pressure of the second formation. The other was his marvelous invention of the wire collar, which also helped the cork withstand the pressure and meant that monks could finally get rid of the iron masks.

The difference in the making of champagne compared to regular wines 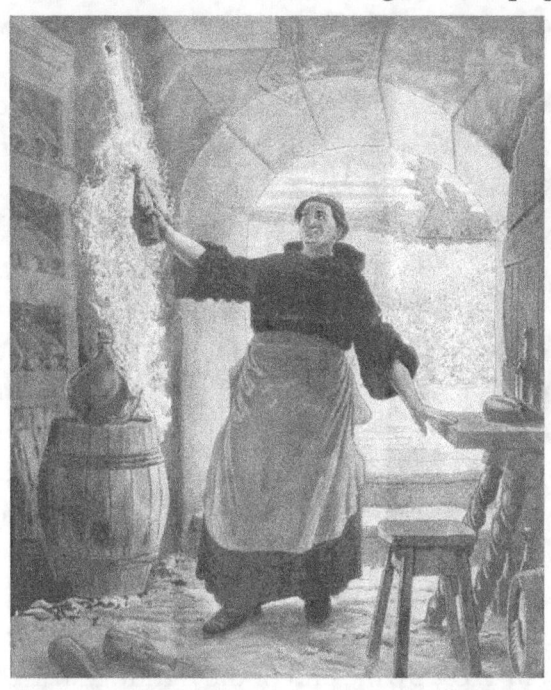 is that there is a second fermentation process, which involves adding several more grams of yeast and then letting it ferment in the bottle. The carbon dioxide produced by this second fermentation then causes the bubbles (of carbon dioxide) to be released rapidly when the bottle is opened, because carbon dioxide is not very soluble.

The champagne at this time was in fact far sweeter than what we drink today; this was because the Russians liked to have at least 300g of sugar per liter. It was not until 1846 when Perrier Jouët decided not to sweeten the champagne before exporting it to England. This led to the trend towards the drier champagnes that we enjoy today.

The Friars of the Catholic Church took wine and wine making to the New World and it wasn't long before Hernando Cortez, as Governor of Mexico in 1525, ordered the planting of grapes. The success was such that the King of Spain forbid new plantings or vineyard replacements in Mexico after 1595, fearing his colony would become self-sufficient in wine. This edict was enforced for 150 years, effectively preventing a commercial wine industry from forming. As in Europe, however, vineyards survived under the auspices of the church and the care of the missions. In 1769, Franciscan missionary Father Junipero Serra planted the first California vineyard at

Mission San Diego. Father Serra continued to establish eight more missions and vineyards until his death in 1784 and has been called the "Father of California Wine". The variety he planted, presumably descended from the original Mexican plantings, became known as the Mission grape and dominated California wine production until about 1880.

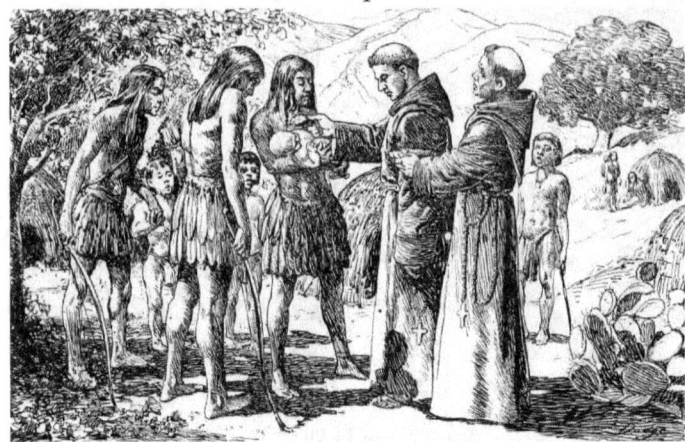

Meanwhile back in France, wine making was still very important. By 1725, Bordeaux had already classified the finest red wines it produced but an official classification based on prices wasn't created until as late as 1855. This classification divided the wines into up to 5 classes or crus.

This all came to an abrupt end at the start of little thing know the world over as The French Revolution in 1789, by the end of the fighting, in 1799, the power was with people and not the King, who had, shall we say, been dispatched. More importantly though, the wine vineyards were in the hands of the common people. The newly founded French Republic removed all feudal privileges that the Catholic Clergy and the nobles possessed.

Any nobles who didn't manage to flee also lost their heads. All of the church and noble land was repossessed and the vineyards were now in the peasants' hands. This was crucial for the development of wine, as now vineyards were in competition and the owners' entire livelihoods depended on the success of the vineyards. This led to the continued growth of the French wine industry, at least until Phylloxera arrived. But more on that in a moment.

Back in the New World, wines such as those from Australia and the Americas were soon to appear. These wines are often looked down upon as inferior to European wine. Although they are now starting to produce some exquisite wines, it must also be said that these countries supply a large amount of standard table wine and less fine wine compared to Europe.

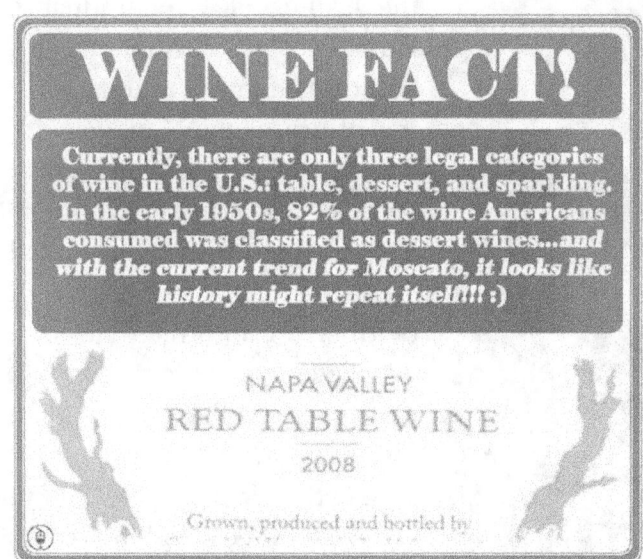

WINE FACT!

Currently, there are only three legal categories of wine in the U.S.: table, dessert, and sparkling. In the early 1950s, 82% of the wine Americans consumed was classified as dessert wines...and with the current trend for Moscato, it looks like history might repeat itself!!! :)

NAPA VALLEY
RED TABLE WINE
2008
Grown, produced and bottled by

Wine was first brought to South America by the Spanish and once again purely for religious reasons. Wine arrived in North America via the colonists fleeing from religious persecution to start a new life in the new world.

Not surprisingly, there were many Catholics in the mix and as I've mentioned before wine is deeply rooted in Catholicism. California is the largest producer of wine in the USA at the moment. The wines in America are named after the grape variety used rather than in France where they, of course, named them after the region of origin.

California's first documented imported European wine vines were planted in Los Angeles in 1833, just some 30 years after the French Revolution, by a Frenchman named Jean-Louis Vignes. In the 1850s and

'60s, the colorful Agoston Harazsthy, a Hungarian soldier, merchant and promoter, made several trips to import cuttings from 165 of the greatest European vineyards to California. Some of this endeavor was at his personal expense and some through grants from the state. Overall, he introduced about 300 different grape varieties, although some were lost prior to testing, due to difficulties in preserving and handling.

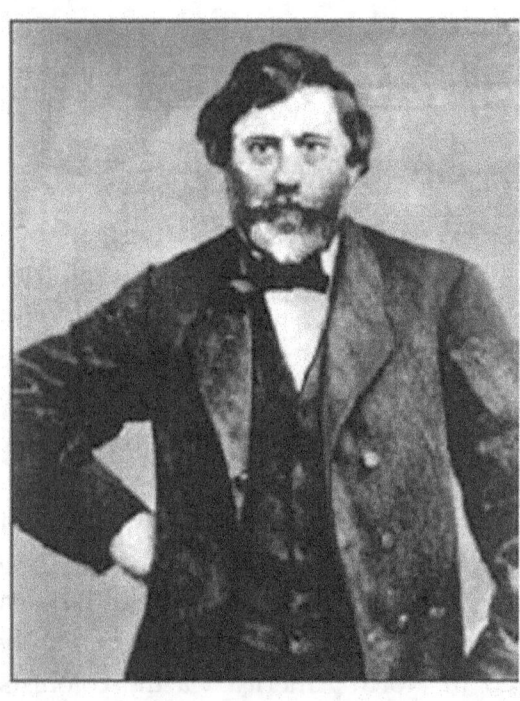

Besides founding Buena Vista winery in 1857, Agoston Haraszthy is credited with founding Sauk City, Wisconsin, serving as the first federal marshall of San Diego, and was posthumously inducted into the Culinary Institute of America's Vintners Hall of Fame earlier this year.

Considered the Founder of the California Wine Industry, Harazsthy contributed his enthusiasm and optimism for the future of wine, along with considerable personal effort and risk. He founded Buena Vista winery and promoted vine planting over much of Northern California. He dug extensive caves for cellaring, promoted hillside planting, fostered the idea of non-irrigated vineyards and suggested Redwood for casks when oak supplies ran low. Initially, wine was shunned as it was thought of as far too European and therefore, not welcome in the newly founded United States of America. Even if they had been keen to make wine, they had little time with which to do so as they were rather busy taming the new world they lived in.

The popularity of wine hasn't grown much and the US public still remain largely beer drinkers. Only 30% of the population have come to realize the far superior experience of wine drinking. Of that 30%, a whopping 75% of the wine they drink is made in America.

As you can see, there is still a slightly isolationist approach to wine in America. Australia had similar problems with producing wine earlier on, as they too were a new country and had even more hostile surroundings to tame.

The only advancement that has been made by these countries is the way they make their oak barrels for the aging fine wine. It was thought that French oak was the best for imparting its flavor into wines. This was mainly because American oaks (as well as oak from many other countries) had been used to make barrels, but the effect of the wood on the wine was far too great or heavy.

It was later discovered that it wasn't the wood that was the problem, but the way the barrels were made. As the Americans were more accustomed to making whiskey barrels they dried their wood in a kiln, unlike the coopers who let their wood air dry for at least 24 months before using. The other difference was that the Americans sawed the wood into staves, whereas the coopers split the wood. These differences to the techniques used immediately made a substantial difference to the wine produced. After this discovery, the Americans and Australians were finally able to start making some quality fine wine. These were perhaps, still not quite as good as the finest French wines, but they were getting there and in the future they would even give the French a run for their money.

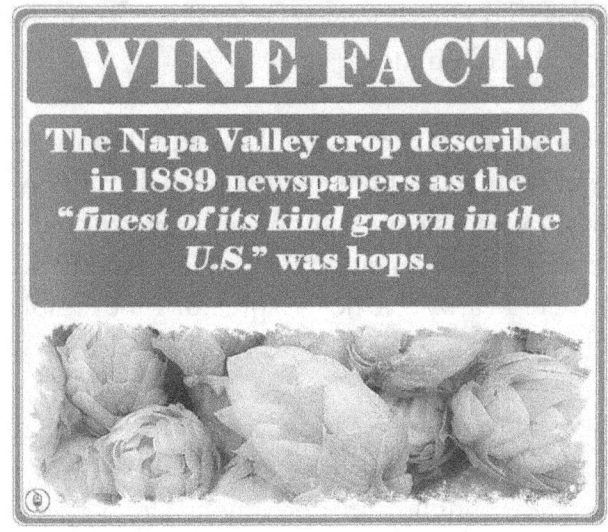

WINE FACT!

The Napa Valley crop described in 1889 newspapers as the "finest of its kind grown in the U.S." was hops.

For centuries wine was produced and enjoyed with little thought for and no true understanding of its underlying science, wine evolved through "spontaneous generation," as far as anyone knew. French chemist Louis Pasteur, among many discoveries relating to his germ theory of diseases, first proposed and proved, in 1857, that wine is made by microscopic organisms, yeasts. This led to the discovery and development of different yeast types and properties and ultimately to better hygiene, less spoilage, and greater efficiency in wine production.

In 1860, Dr. Jules Guyot, another Frenchman, published the first of three treatises describing regional traditional vinicultural and viticultural practices as well as his own observations and arguments on the economy of grape growing. Before these documents, viniculture was a practice that had been apprenticed from generation to generation for over 4000 years, with very few written records and no formal instruction.

In 1863, species of native American grapes were taken to Botanical Gardens in England. These cuttings carried a species of root louse called *phylloxera vastatrix* which attacks and feeds on the vine roots and leaves. Phylloxera is indigenous to the Mississippi River Valley and was unknown outside North America at the time. Powdery mildew, a fungal disease, also indigenous to North America, had previously migrated to Europe and caused problems in some areas. No one, however, had any idea of the wide-reaching destructive potential of Phylloxera.

Native American varieties developed resistance to phylloxera by evolving a thick and tough root bark, so that they were relatively immune to damage. The vinifera vines had no such evolutionary protection and phylloxera ate away at their roots, causing them to rot and the plant to die and driving the pests to seek other nearby live hosts, spreading inexorably through entire vineyards and on to others.

By 1865, phylloxera had spread to vines in Provence. Over the next 20 years, it inhabited and decimated nearly all the vineyards of Europe. Many methods were attempted to eradicate phylloxera: flooding, where possible, and injecting the soil with carbon bisulfide, had some success in checking the louse, but were costly and the pests came back as soon as the treatments stopped.

Finally, Thomas V Munson, a horticulturist from Denison, Texas, realized that native American vines were resistant and suggested grafting the *vinifera* vines onto *riparia* hybrid rootstocks. So, there began a long, laborious process of grafting every wine vine in Europe over to American rootstocks. It was only in this manner that the European wine industry could be retrieved from near extinction. Downy mildew, another fungal disease in American 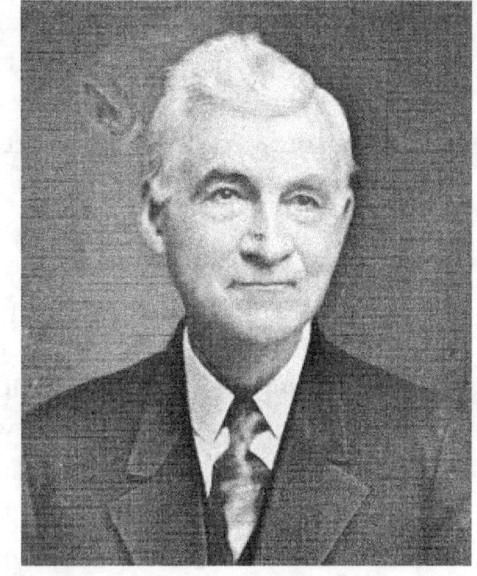 grapevines, unfortunately probably migrated to Europe on some of the rootstocks imported for grafting. One tragic consequence of the Phylloxera devastation is that many of the native species indigenous to Europe, since they were of negligible commercial value, were not perpetuated by grafting and became extinct.

There was some debate generated by this replanting that the quality declined in "post-phylloxera" wines. Whether this was indeed the case and whether this was due to the rootstocks themselves or to the relatively sudden and nearly universal youth of the vines, or to changes in vinification techniques, or to some other concurrent factor or variable, is unknown. Undoubtedly, it will remain a matter of theory and opinion and provide animated conversation at wine tastings, but ultimately never be proven.

European consumer demand was unabated, especially in France, yet the vineyard blights resulted in shortages of wine for many years. French producers turned their focus to the French North African colonies of

Morocco, Tunisia, and particularly Algeria. Fraud and adulteration became problems. In a short period of just over a decade, Algeria grew into the World's largest wine exporter, taking over the position of France. As their industry gradually recovered, ultimately it was competition from these African colonies that spurred French wine growers to the form the system of Appellation Controlée. AC became the model for all wine producing countries to both protect reputations and markets for the wine trade and authenticate product origins for consumers.

During the period when the Europeans were contending with phylloxera, the American wine industry was ironically flourishing. By 1900, America had a fully developed and proud commercial wine producing business. Leading brands from California, New York, Ohio, Missouri, Texas and New Jersey were appearing on many of the best restaurant wine lists alongside French, German and Italian listings. Barrels of California wine were being regularly exported to Australia, Canada, Central America, England, Germany, Mexico and the Orient.

The destruction of the American wine industry would come not from an entomological pest, but from a political one. While it took a hundred years instead of 20 to complete its course, the results were even more devastating. It didn't spread from 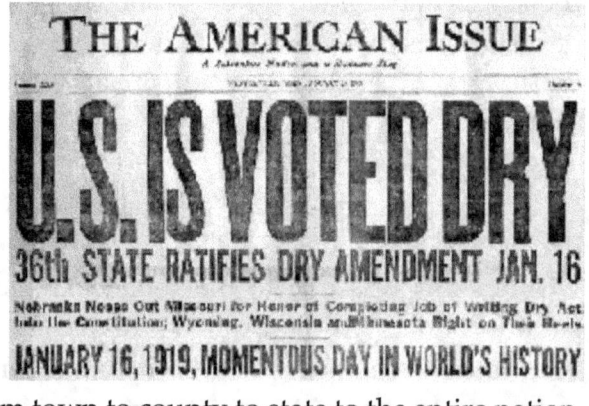 vineyard to vineyard, but from town to county to state to the entire nation.

Alcohol abuse and alcoholism and their related problems were much more widespread and affected a radically larger share of America's population in the early and mid-1800s than they do today. Excessive use, rather than moderate use, was the norm in an era of fewer entertainments and diversions.

The first Prohibition law went on the books in Indiana in 1816, forbidding the sale of any alcohol on Sunday (still enforced to this day). By the 1840s, many towns and counties in Georgia, Indiana, Iowa, Michigan, New Hampshire, New York and Ohio had gone legally "dry". In 1851, Maine enacted the first statewide law prohibiting the manufacture and sale of liquor and, by 1855, thirteen of the thirty-one United States had followed suit.

The Industrial Revolution led from local to large-scale brewing and mass marketing, with intense competition. A proliferation of saloons drove owners to seek side profits by pursuing illegal and unsavory vices such as gambling and prostitution. As another beverage containing alcohol, wine began to suffer the successful excesses of beer.

In 1880, Kansas became the first state to go "dry" by amending their Constitution, followed by Iowa, Georgia, Oklahoma, Mississippi, North Carolina, Tennessee, West Virginia and Virginia. Although some of these laws allowed winemaking to continue for sale elsewhere, few wineries in these states could compete without selling their wines locally. Most closed their doors and abandoned their vineyards.

The Drys went so far as to have any mention of wine expunged from school and college texts, including Greek and Roman classic literature. Medicinal wines were dropped from the United States Pharmacopoeia. They even tried to prove that praises for wine in the Bible were actually referring to unfermented grape juice. Thirty-three states had gone dry at the outbreak of World War I.

In December, 1917, Congress passed the Eighteenth Amendment to the U.S. Constitution, criminalizing the "manufacture, sale, or transportation of intoxicating liquors"; by February, 1919, 45 states had ratified it; New Jersey held out until 1922, and only Connecticut and Rhode Island ultimately rejected it. To define the language and set the effective date, Congress enacted the National Prohibition Act, more popularly known as the Volstead Act, named after Minnesota Republican Andrew Volstead, tee-totaler and primary proponent of the bill. After midnight on January 16, 1920, National Prohibition would begin.

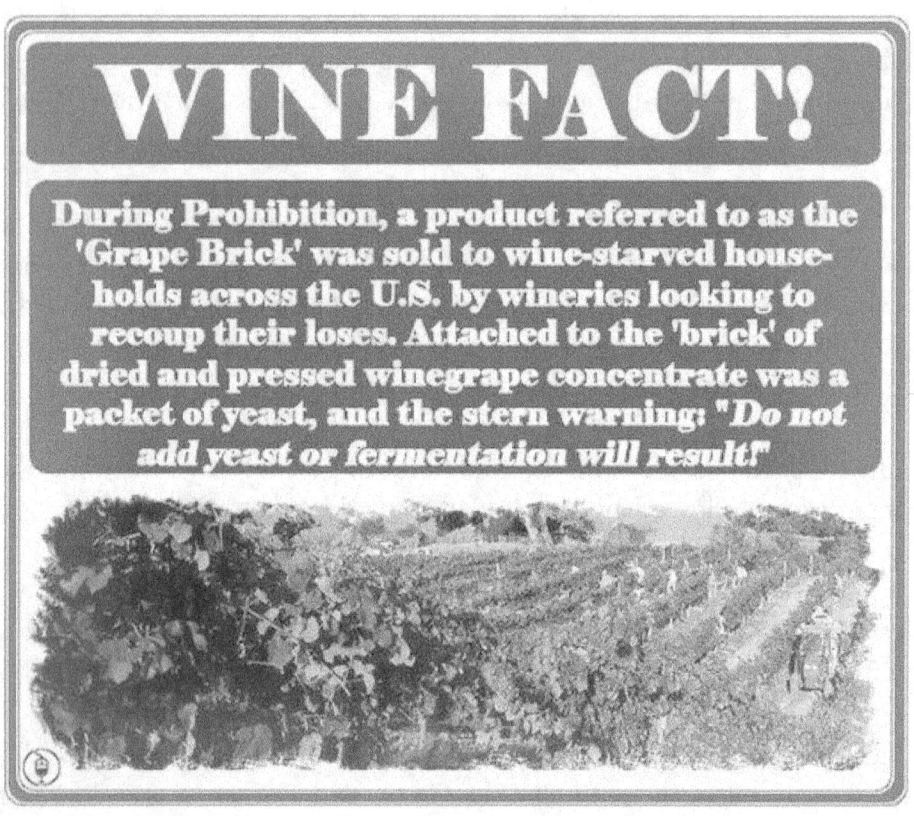

WINE FACT!

During Prohibition, a product referred to as the 'Grape Brick' was sold to wine-starved households across the U.S. by wineries looking to recoup their loses. Attached to the 'brick' of dried and pressed winegrape concentrate was a packet of yeast, and the stern warning: *"Do not add yeast or fermentation will result!"*

The net consequences of the legislation made it much more difficult to obtain alcohol, possession by individuals for personal consumption was not a federal crime. Through a provision that made penalties not applicable to "a person manufacturing nonintoxicating cider and fruit juice exclusively for use in his home," thousands of otherwise law-abiding citizens became home winemaking hobbyists and quasi-bootleggers. This poorly-constructed clause eliminated punishments without strictly legalizing either home brewing or winemaking, yet the obvious difficulty of interpreting and applying the law's intent led to new pastimes for many households.

Explosive demand for fresh grapes and a shortage of refrigerated railroad cars in which to ship them caused prices to skyrocket. Growers began replanting their vineyards from fine wine varieties over to table or juice grape varieties that shipped better. Planted acreage nearly doubled from 1919 to 1926. Vineyard land prices climbed from $200 an acre in 1918 to $2,500 an acre in 1923. Prosperity for the growers lasted barely five years. In 1925, the railroads finally had enough cars, too much fruit was shipped and it rotted on the Eastern docks. In 1926, vineyard land fell back to $250 per acre. The massive plantings produced a constant surplus of California grapes that persisted until 1971.

By the time of National Repeal, effective December 5, 1933, the industry was in ruins. Although some wineries managed to survive by obtaining permits to make wines used for medicinal, sacramental and non-beverage additive purposes, production dropped 94% from 1919 to 1925.

Health Benefits of Red Wine

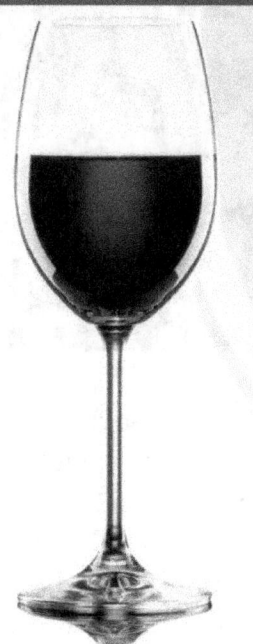

Rich in diuretic properties

Boosts resistance to allergens

Prevents cancer and heart diseases

Helps prevent diabetes and hypertension

Reduces risk of gallstones and kidney stones

Beneficial in slowing down the aging process

Reduces risk of dementia and Alzheimer's disease

Even after Repeal, several states stayed dry: Kansas until 1948, Oklahoma until 1957, and Mississippi until 1966. Seventeen states chose to obliterate free-market capitalism by establishing monopoly liquor stores with limited selections and plain-as-dirt merchandising that discourages "respectable" housewives from shopping.

There remain local prohibitions that are arbitrary, inconsistent and niggling, with such manifest foolishness as streets lined door-to-door on one side with taverns and "package stores" and nary a one on the opposite side where the dry boundary runs down the middle of the roadway. Today 10 percent of the nation's area and 6 percent of the population remain dry.

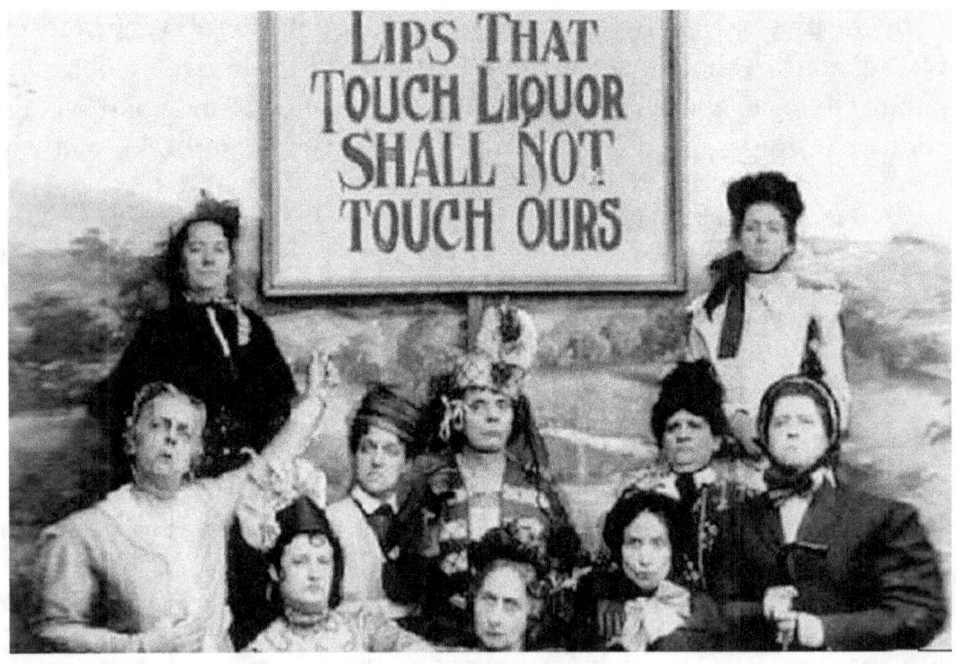

Anticipating Repeal, speculators and quick-buck artists soon flooded the legal market with quickly and poorly made wine. Dilettantes published books and articles warning Americans about rigid rules that must be followed to serve the proper wine with the proper food from the proper glass at the proper temperature. Faced with bad-tasting products with which to risk committing social blunders and while remaining uncertain about the social acceptance of any alcohol, most Americans stayed away. Hard drinkers stuck to hard liquor. For decades, moderate wine drinking in a social context survived almost exclusively in households that made their own.

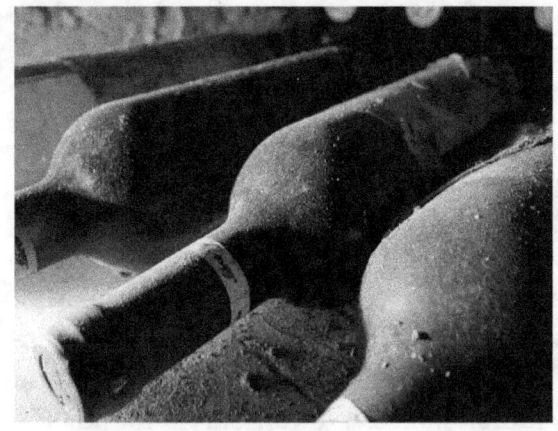

The only group of wines that sold well following Repeal were the fortified dessert wines. Taxed at the lower rate of wine as opposed to distilled spirits, but with 20 percent alcohol, this group made the cheapest intoxicant available for derelicts and winos. Recovery and re-growth of the American wine industry was severely inhibited for the next half century, in both quantity and quality.

Before 1920, there were more than 2,500 commercial wineries in the United States. Less than 100 survived as winemaking operations to 1933. By 1960, that number had grown to only 271. California had 713 bonded wineries before Prohibition; it took more than half a century, until 1986, before that many were again operating.

Before 1920, table wines accounted for 3 of every 4 gallons shipped. In 1937, four years after Repeal, fortified wine production outpaced table wine by a ratio of 5 to 1. It wasn't until 1968 that table wines sales caught up and finally overtook fortified wines, regaining the status of most popular wine category.

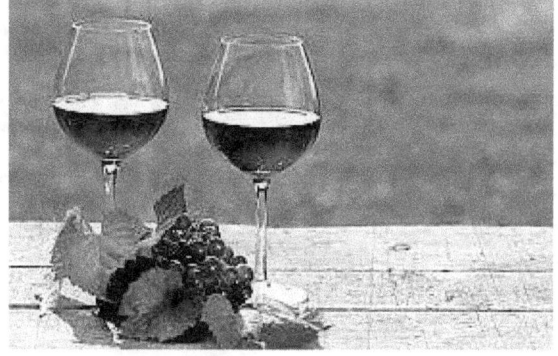

Prohibition left a legacy of distorting the role of alcohol in American life, ruining a fledgling world-class wine industry, weakening the U.S. Constitution, and boosting the success and profitability of Organized Crime (the price of whiskey rose over 500% during the 1920s). The maze of confusing and conflicting laws that currently vary widely between states impedes commerce, sustains distribution monopolies, casts aspersions of greed on tax coffers, and mocks the American sense of fair competition.

More police officers were killed during the decade of the 1920s than in any decade in history. The "Grand Experiment" implanted moral ambiguity and disrespect for authority in an entire generation of Americans, while it deprived them of potential social and health benefits, and brought the character and term "wino" into the streets and the lexicon. The one positive remainder is the lingering Congressional hesitance to pass Constitutional Amendments, especially regarding restrictions on individual liberty and personal moral choice. We can only hope for the future that our representatives don't commit such folly when powerful special interests clash with the shared individual freedoms that make up the public interest.

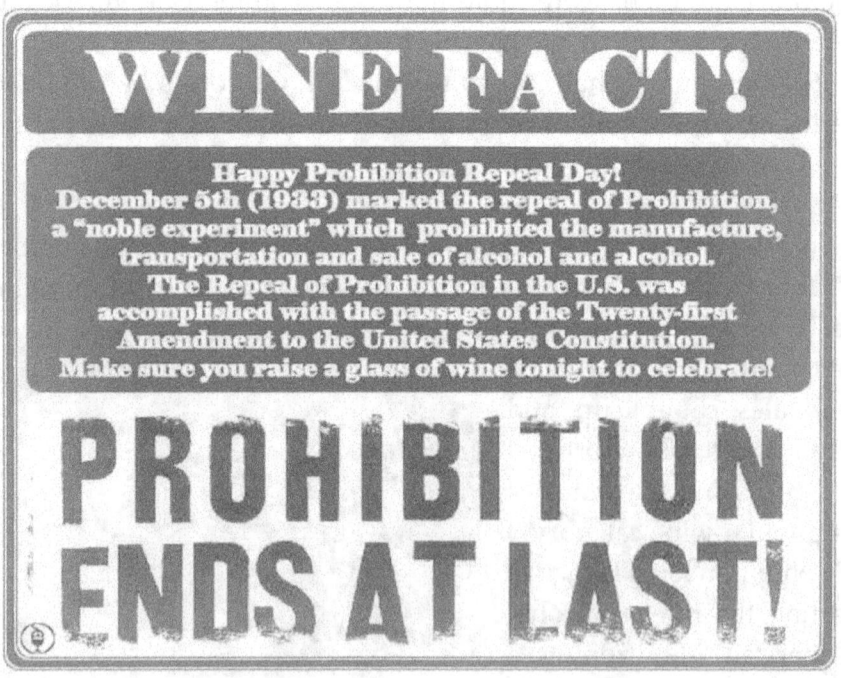

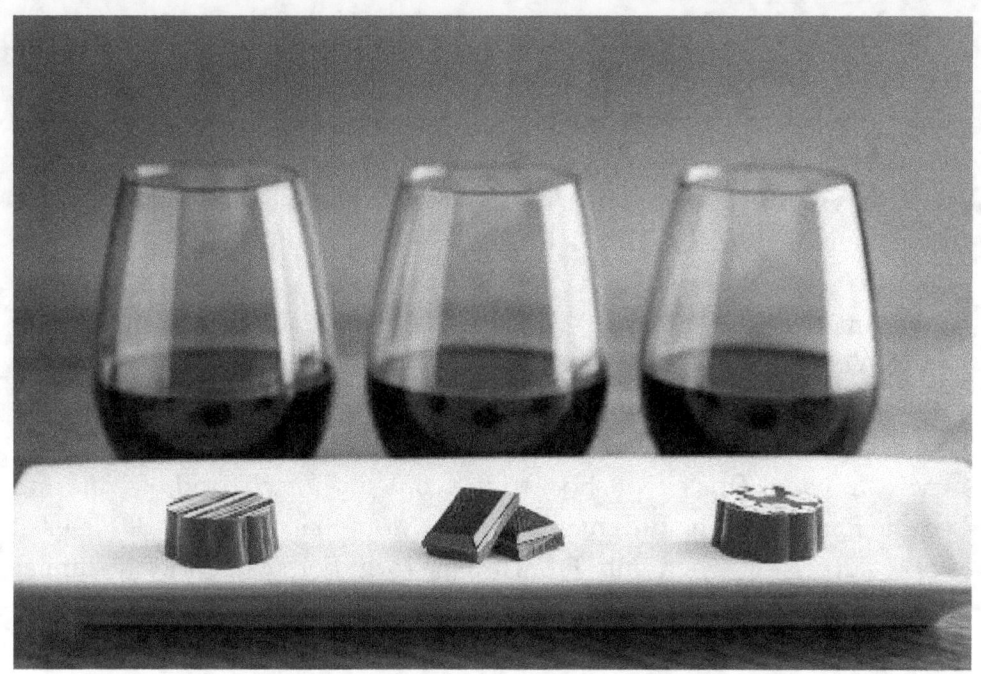

The forces of prohibition are not dead yet. They are more insidious, combining moralist and monopolist factions, pursuing an agenda of obstructionist legislation, that includes preventing or encumbering direct sales of wine to consumers, preventing health information from being printed on wine labels and spreading disinformation about potential benefits and studies related to wine and health.

In spite of the political workings, table wine grew in popularity in America during the last half of the 20th Century. U.S. per-capita consumption of wine still lags far behind most countries of the Western Hemisphere. American wine-consuming growth is on pace to become the number one wine consuming nation by 2020.

A remaining problem is American tendency toward excess. More than 85% of the volume of wine America drinks is done by less than 8% of the total population. A goal of moderate regular consumption seems too tame for America's tastes. Achieving such might bring better health overall to the population and peace with all but the most radical tee-totalers.

Research in the past thirty years has led to developments in both agriculture and technology that have greatly improved overall wine quality. The quality and stature of California and other American wine has never been better and worldwide demand continues to grow. The attractions of the "gentleman farming" lifestyle and the increasing demand drove the industry to swell to a total of 4,383 bonded US wineries in 2006.

In America's Bicentennial Year of 1976, two California wines (Stag's Leap Wine Cellars 1973 Estate Cabernet Sauvignon and Chateau Montelena 1973 Napa Valley Chardonnay) bested their top French wine counterparts at a blind tasting in Paris judged entirely by Frenchmen, all experts in wine! This event shocked the contemporary world of wine and became famous as The Judgment of Paris. More than four decades later, it is now surprising when only French wines win both categories at similar events.

In the 21st Century we are fortunate to live in a world in which both good table wines and a wide and growing selection of fine wines are produced in wineries all over the world!

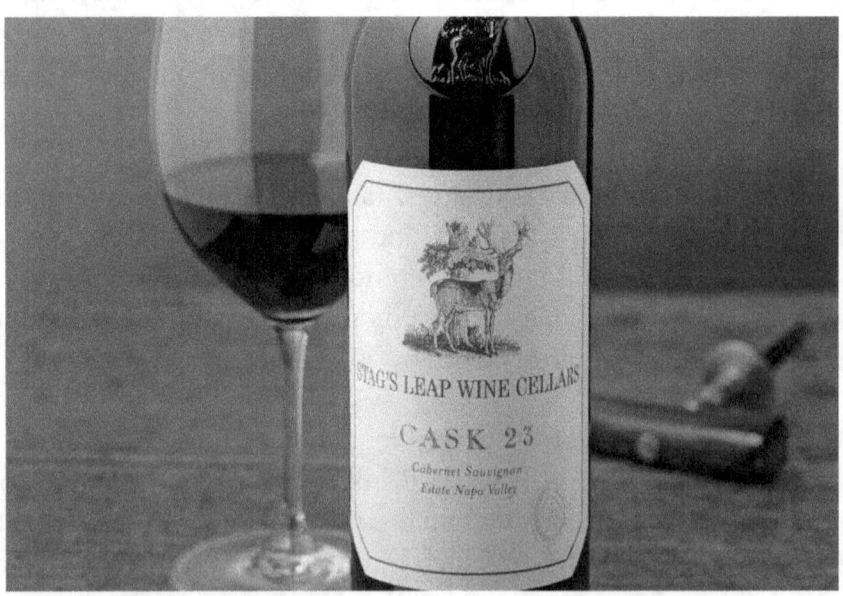

6. Yes, Food IS Medicine!

"Let food be thy medicine and medicine be thy food." This quote is attributed to Hippocrates. Another of my favorite quotes is *"Who said anything about medicine? Let's eat!"* which is attributed to one of Hippocrates forgotten (and hilarious) students.

Who hasn't seen or heard Hippocrates' famous quote above? If you have Facebook friends who are the least bit into "natural" medicine or living, you've almost certainly come across it in your feed, and if you're a reader of my Phytonutrient Blog, you will absolutely have heard the quote. Now, Hippocrates lived a very long time ago, that is definitely true but just because an idea is old, doesn't mean it's good, any more than just because Hippocrates said it means it must be true. But in this case, it does and it is!

Remember, Hippocrates was an important figure in the history of medicine because he was among the earliest to assert that diseases were caused by natural processes rather than the gods and because of his emphasis on the careful observation and documentation of patient history and physical findings, which led to the discovery of physical signs associated with diseases of specific organs. He is also known to have been a great healer because of his knowledge of the culinary and medicinal uses of herbs and spices.

But you know what? Hippocrates was not the only advocate for letting food be thy medicine. Throughout the ages there have been many others. Ever since man first climbed down from the trees (or, depending upon your view, plucked that apple off that tree), eating has never been far from his mind (survival has a way of prioritizing everything). The simple fact that sustenance equals life, means that food and health have culturally ridden shotgun throughout the ages.

"Good men eat and drink so they can live," noted Socrates.

"Eat, drink, and be merry!" commanded Solomon.

"You're famished. I'll fix you a plate!!" pleaded my mother. And, most likely, yours too.

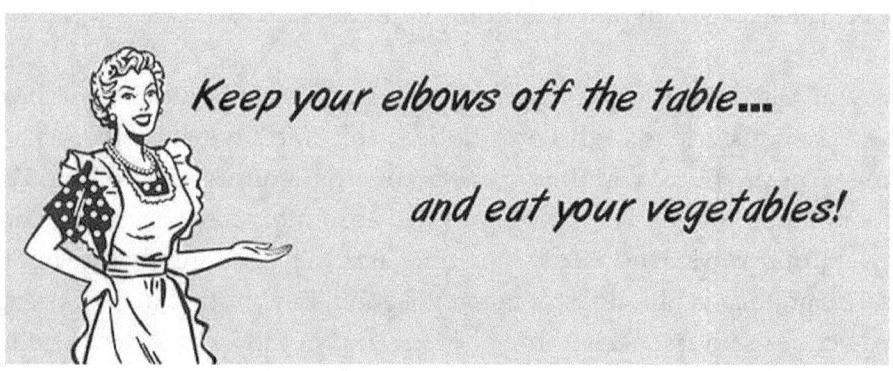

In the days before medicine, food was medicine…or at least it was seen as such. A browned apple for an upset stomach, chicken soup for congestion, champagne for septicemia (Pulitzer Prize-winning novelist Eudora Welty said her Mississippi father swore his use of the bubbly saved her ill mother's life). It was sometimes hard to establish cause and effect (Garlic as an anti-vampiric? Hard to find test subjects for that one,) and yet generations of pantries held foods sworn to bind, purge, ameliorate, instigate, invigorate…in short, improve one's well-being.

And then came modern allopathic-oriented science, which until recently tossed nutrition—and its potential effect on both maintaining health and calming illness—into the compost heap. The reasons were myriad. Politically, no one had ever been elected on an anti-cheeseburger platform, so administrative pressure to funnel government dollars toward nutritional research traditionally was nil. Similarly, big pharma was scarce with cash, because they can't patent a food's natural properties. And from a practical viewpoint, studying food with its thousands of chemicals and nutrients is incredibly complex. By comparison, targeting and studying a single drug for efficacy in a double-blind model was far more straightforward and lucrative to both researchers and industry.

It took the American Medical Association until 2002 to reverse a long-standing position and suggest that adults take a multivitamin every day. Then again, many of its long-standing members had never been exposed to a nutrition elective while in medical school...creating a drug-oriented bias that historically expressed itself in both the clinic and the lab.

"I think for a long time the major directions in molecular biology—the ability to make genetically altered mice that could measure the impacts of certain molecules on the body—was totally not applied to nutrition," - Hopkins' William Nelson, director of the Sidney Kimmel Cancer Center.

That Nelson can speak of such research deficiencies in the past tense is indicative of a huge shift toward nutritional research in just the past 10 to 15 years. Again I remind you that the information I present in this series, while in truth very old is now being backed by 21st Century science and research!

What then is the catalyst for this paradigm shift in thinking?

Well since you asked I'll tell you what I think. We can't seem to shut our mouths, and the stats from the Centers for Disease Control back that up! With the exception of Colorado dwellers, more than 20% of the U.S. population is now considered obese. Given obesity's epidemiologically supported impact on cardiac, vascular, cancer, and diabetic-related illness, researchers are now branching out to uncover the myriad ways food and its micro components enhance or disrupt life. The sheer numbers of nutritional studies bear out this interest. According to Pub Med, such published investigations more than doubled between the 1980s and 1990s, and leapt another 71% this decade. Part of the quantum leap in the last five years especially, is the discovery that chronic inflammation is slowly being linked to diseases including cancer, and that foods—from cloves to walnuts—appear to contain anti-inflammatory properties.

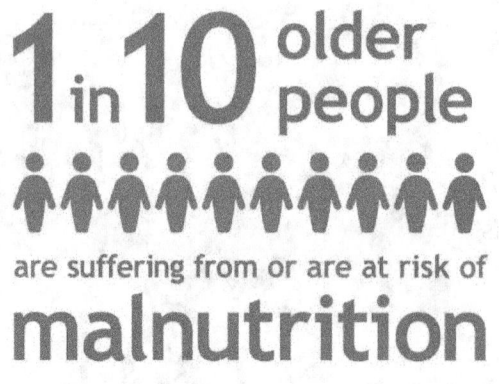

This critical mass of information even has a name. Called the 'Food as Medicine movement', it's a growing recognition on the part of many academic clinicians that to ignore the role of food and nutrition in health is to lose a valuable tool that can support (or perhaps even lessen or replace) many pharmaceuticals currently in use.

"The perfect example is ginger," says Hopkins gastroenterologist Gerard Mullin, arguably the nation's top expert on the relationship between food and gut disorders. *"People who have nausea, or gastric dysmotilities or other GI problems, for them ginger is at the top of my list. It works the same way (the big pharma produced) Zofran does, which is*

one of our most powerful anti-nausea drugs. It works on the same receptor in the brain. But a lot of docs aren't aware of it."

Similarly, food plays a huge role in how well people battle cancer. Researchers estimate that some 80% of cancer patients are malnourished, at the very time when chemotherapy often increases the body's need for proteins and other nutrients. Such malnourishment, if not addressed, can lead to a reduction of chemotherapy doses and ultimately poorer outcomes. Oncologist Bill Nelson says that the link between the amount of calories taken in—the so-called "caloric budget"—and its relationship to cancer is of great interest to him. Nelson notes that caloric intake drops among the elderly, while their cancer rates rise. It may well be that taking in fewer calories—especially of food of little to no nutritional value—leaves elders deprived of nutrients they need to stave off cancer, he says.

The thirst for nutritional knowledge is by no means limited to physicians and wellness professionals. A poll of attendees of A Women's Journey, an annual women's health symposium sponsored by Hopkins Medicine, showed a huge demand for more seminars devoted to the nuances of nutrition, and faculty speakers who could make sense of the flood of dietary data being unleashed on the public.

In response, the Fall 2009 A Woman's Journey featured numerous talks with a nutritional component, including three seminars—led by the aforementioned Nelson, Mullin, and nutritionist Lynda McIntyre—that, like a well-balanced meal, triangulated how different research approaches are translating into smarter ways to eat for health. For Gerard Mullin, nutrition and health have always been intertwined. What's different now is the scientific rigor being applied to the field.

"My mom had the first health food store in northern New Jersey. I've cooked since I was 10," says Mullin. *"I was raised on food as medicine, and I'm glad the science has really borne out and supported what many of us were raised to believe since we were yay high."*

Mullin refers to himself as an integrative gastroenterologist, the adjective referring to physicians who use complementary modalities including stress management and nutrition in their clinical practices. In both interviews and talks, Mullin lays out a compelling explanation for the mind/body connection to the gut, and how different foods, spices, and herbs can promote better digestive health, especially in the 90 million Americans suffering from digestive diseases.

He focuses on the common negative feedback loop affecting the "cephalic" phase of digestion—the gastric and saliva secretions that occur when appetite is stimulated but before eating actually begins. Sleep deprivation, emotional upset, poor eating habits—all can lead to an impaired cephalic phase. It's the stomach's equivalent of not being in the mood, and the response is somewhat the same. Diminished blood flow impairs function: In this case the gut doesn't absorb nutrients. All that unabsorbed food can make us miserable (i.e., everything from diarrhea to gas, bloating, and beyond). That jacks up stress levels, makes eating even more undesirable, and before you know it you've worked yourself into a case of irritable bowel syndrome or worse.

While drugs can treat symptoms, Mullin says breaking the cycle is both a mental and physical process. Taking the time to cook can in itself enhance that first cephalic phase—everything from the meditative act of chopping to inhaling rich aromas can be relaxing—while choosing certain foods such as peppermint leaves and ground flax may reduce gut spasms.

According to British Medical Journal studies, Mullin says, *"Peppermint works better than most IBS drugs. It works on relaxing calcium channel blockers. Sometimes it can make your gut so relaxed, right between the gut and esophagus, that you get some burping or heartburn, so you have to be careful how much you use. More isn't always better."*

At Hopkins, Mullin has worked to improve both nutrition and timely access to food given to Johns Hopkins Hospital inpatients.

"In a hospital setting, anywhere from 33% to 55% of people are malnourished," he notes.

With study funding from Department of Medicine Chief Mike Weisfeldt, says Mullin, "we proved that if you feed people earlier (following admission), their hospital stay is shorter and outcome is much better. It is common sense, but we had to show the evidence.

1 in 3 people aged 65+ are at risk of malnutrition on admission to hospital

And it's reawakened a whole discussion" about improving gut health through diet.

Mullin notes that many common kitchen staples can be very effective for preventing and relieving gut-related maladies.

"Caraway has been well-studied," Mullin says. *"Its oil is a treatment for gastroparesis, so for those with slow motility and problems with their upper GI tract, caraway can promote motility. Fennel, ginger, dill, cumin...all these things can help you on an everyday basis."*

From both a taste and nutrient viewpoint, fresh is generally better than dried, though dried is better than nothing. As for amounts, most research suggests moderation as a key, the idea being that it's the continuous, sustainable addition of herbs and other nutrients that enhance flavor and long-term gut health. Do not skip meals, eating regularly and including herbs and spices, fruit and vegetables, and fish is truly necessary to optimum health especially in our young and elderly.

Equally important is what foods to avoid. Improving that cephalic response will be pretty much a waste if the gut is being overdosed with junk. Mullin cites studies noting that, while the average American consumes 100 grams of fructose a day—everything from "soda to ketchup to grapes"—the body can only tolerate about 50 grams. The overload acts as an IBS and gas trigger.

22% of people aged 60+ skipped meals

to cut back on food costs

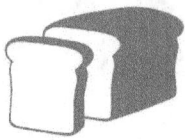

"The first thing we do is say, 'Look, if you want to get better, you have to find a way to eliminate some of these sugars." He says.

Mullin aims his last culinary salvo at inflammation. Many scientists believe that certain aspects of lifestyle—notably what we eat—can create a chronic inflammatory state within cells, tissues, and organs. In short, the immune system is in constant attack mode, which may have deleterious effects on health.

"We know that many conditions in the gut are mediated through inflammation. We're appreciating that now more than ever," he says, pointing to recent research links. *"How do you help make yourself better? Again, it's a food as medicine approach. There are (anti-inflammatory) studies about blueberries and blackberries out there (see "Allies in the Pantry.")*

Bill Nelson's interest in food literally comes down to a flip of the wrist. No, not as a chef, but rather a scientist fascinated by how foods—notably meats—are altered by the way they're cooked. Using World Health Organization data, Nelson concluded that some 35% of cancers probably include a dietary element, with inflammation—which could also have dietary factors—playing a role in perhaps another 30% of cases.

A highly respected molecular biologist and cancer clinician—he's principal investigator for one of the National Cancer Institute's Specialized Program of Research Excellence (SPORE) initiatives—Nelson has taken a microscopic interest in the interplay of diet and prostate cancer.

He notes that not only do Asian men have far less prostate cancer than their American counterparts, they appear far less prone to inflammation.

When comparing autopsies of non-cancerous prostates of men who live in America versus those in Asia,

"Every prostate removed here showed signs of inflammation, while the Asian prostates were pristine." Curiously, the longer Asian men are in America, the more likely they are to develop prostate cancer. *"If they're here 25 years or more, their rate becomes half that of Caucasians, and if their kids are born here, their risk is the same as Caucasians. There must be something in the lifestyle risks that we can reduce."*

While Asians tend to eat far more fish and far less meat and fowl than Americans, Nelson says that might not tell the whole story. The problem may lie in how we heat our meats.

"Heat changes a huge amount of the components in food," says Nelson, focusing on two particular carcinogens that can be created by cooking. The first, called heterocyclic amines, are formed by the heat-catalyzed interplay between creatinine (found in the muscle of meats and fish) and amino acids.

One heterocyclic amine called "PhIP" is extremely nasty: When given to rats in doses comparable to those consumed by humans, the male rats rapidly developed prostate and colon cancer, while the female rats developed colon and breast cancer.

"For us, that was fascinating," recalled Nelson. *"We just said, 'Holy cow! It is incredible that something you could eat could do that."*

Not only can the amount and duration of heat increase these dangerous amines (i.e., well-done appears worse for you than medium or medium rare), but so

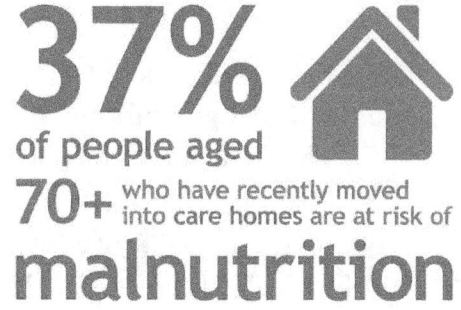

37% of people aged **70+** who have recently moved into care homes are at risk of **malnutrition**

can cooking technique. *"You can take burger patties, put them on the same skillet, control for temperature and time, but in one case you flip them only once, in the middle of cooking, while the other you flip every 30 seconds."* The burgers only flipped once *"make a ton of amines,"* notes Nelson. *"So did sausages cooked as links versus patties."* The links, in Nelson's opinion, act *"as closed reaction vessels."* Nelson's own research uncovered that in many cases the liver can't metabolize all these "charred" meat carcinogens, and passes them through to the prostate, where people with a particular DNA mutation may be at much higher risk for developing cancer.

Nelson also points out that the fat dripping along a deep grilled steak might taste delicious, but it's potentially deadly. The culprit, which also escapes from the fat in chicken skin, is something called polycyclic aromatic hydrocarbon carcinogens. To put some numbers to the science, Nelson says the amount of these carcinogens consumed daily by the average American *"equals ingesting half a pack of cigarette smoke a day."*

My suggestion: **If you're going to eat meat, stick to lower-fat cuts, take the skin off of chicken before cooking, and look at alternatives such as broiling or, in the case of fish, poaching the filet. Remember too that fat in the diet is important, but it is the right fats – like olive oil or the fats that are found in fish that we need – not a ton of beef or poultry fats.**

Nelson believes that both the public and industry are ready to hear his message. In meetings with executives at a large grocery store, Nelson discovered that 16% of the chain's sales came from pre-cooked foods and meals that busy customers quickly reheated at home. The executives had quite an appetite for Nelson's food prep science. Not only would such techniques improve food safety, but long term, the executives saw such preparatory expertise as potentially marketable to health-conscious consumers.

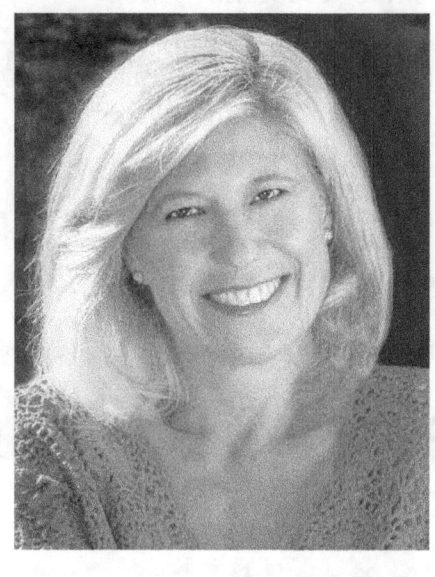

"I'm tantalized about the way we could affect broad-based cooking practices," says Nelson. *"We're at the dawn of an era of figuring this out."*

Figuring out how to translate serious science into tasty, healthy snacks and meals is where nutritionist Lynda McIntyre excels. A registered dietitian with a specialty counseling cancer patients at both the Kimmel Cancer Center at Hopkins and the Sibley Hospital Center for Breast Health in Washington D.C., McIntyre took A Woman's Journey attendees on a virtual tour of the supermarket. Along the way, she busted some myths regarding what it is about food that links it to perhaps the majority of cancer cases.

"A lot of times people think I'm talking about pesticides or additives in food, when in fact I'm not," she says. *"Less than 2% percent of all cancers can be directly related to what the additives are in food. Up to 60 percent can be related to what we're not eating."*

<u>Read that quote again</u> – I know that we are all concerned about pesticides in our food, as we should be, but we need to be at least equally concerned about what **we are and are not eating!** As in enough fruits and vegetables. A familiar message, yes, but McIntyre gives it a twist, suggesting shoppers take a colorful approach to solving their qualms about which produce has the greatest overall benefits. You have heard me say it and now this doctor stresses it too,

"Eat the rainbow. The brighter the food, the richer the color, the higher its anti-oxidant count," counsels McIntyre, who also served on a statewide council that developed cancer prevention strategies for Maryland.

For McIntyre and other savvy nutritionists, the state of food science has allowed them to fine-tune their message and take some of the confusion out of the game. Take fresh versus frozen produce. McIntyre says both are effective…

"Fresh is always best when it is in season," says McIntyre, since fresh produce retains top flavor and nutritional value. However, McIntyre notes that many fresh foods have relatively short seasons. As an alternative, from a nutritional viewpoint, *"frozen can be just as nutritious because it's picked at the peak of ripeness, and frozen to keep the nutritional content intact."*

Then there's eating whole foods versus taking supplements, a source of huge debate. The prevailing sentiment among many researchers is that supplementation can bring someone deficient in a given nutrient up to a supportive baseline, but people already at solid baseline levels may not benefit from additional dosing.

93% of malnourished older people are in the **community.**

"In some cases, single supplementation of antioxidants can increase the risk of certain diseases," says McIntyre. *"For example, vitamin E and heart disease. Another example is that single supplementation of vitamin A can increase bone fractures in women. And in smokers who took beta-carotene, we saw an increase in lung cancer. The studies show it is the whole foods (and how they work together synergistically) that provides the most protective effect to the body."*

Knowing how to combine those foods can increase the body's ability to absorb their nutrients. McIntyre says putting broccoli (sulforaphane) and tomatoes (lycopene) together *"increases their tumor protective ability."* Similarly, carrots and avocado are a nice dynamic duo because beta-carotene is better absorbed in the presence of a fat (short on avocados? Try olive oil). Apples and blueberries, even spinach and strawberries (*"It's a strange combination, but delicious,"* insists McIntyre) all make for nutrient-dense dynamic duos.

So, bottom line, what I want, and need, for you to understand is this; as for the thinking that healthy eating and drinking is restrictive, forget it. Nearly every family of food and beverage that I have researched—be it nut, fruit, spice, fish, grain, beans, chocolate, wine, or beer—has some (often many) members in it filled with high nutritional content. On every conceivable front, from the molecular level to the kitchen table research is unlocking the power of certain foods to keep us in fighting shape. Since none of us has a "foodprint" yet—a DNA or some other molecular roadmap that will tell us why Sally's system can absorb beta-carotene from carrots, while Sue's can only assimilate that same beta-carotene from sweet potatoes—for now, eating a well-rounded, well-informed diet is all about playing the odds. And there's nothing better than improving your chances of beating the house.

So, the next time that someone tries to tell you that you shouldn't eat that chocolate, or that you should lay off of the beer and wine – just tell them that they shouldn't worry, you are just working on improving your health!

If you want more information about this subject check out my *"Yes, Food IS Medicine"* series. It is available at bookstores everywhere or online at Amazon.com. This series was originally published under the title *"Phytonutrient Gardening"* but since so many people did not understand just what the term 'Phytonutrient' meant, my publishers suggested we rebrand the series under the title *"Yes, Food IS Medicine"*. I am so glad that we did! Under the new title the sales of the books has really increased and the word is getting out to people like never before! It is very gratifying.

The **_"Yes, Food IS Medicine"_** series currently is planned to be a four-part collection with the first 3 books already available:

Yes, Food IS Medicine – Book 1: Vegetables

Yes, Food IS Medicine – Book 2: Fruits, Nuts and Seeds

Yes, Food IS Medicine – Book 3: Herbs and Spices

Yes, Food IS Medicine – Book 4: Teas and Wild Edibles

(coming in the fall of 2017)

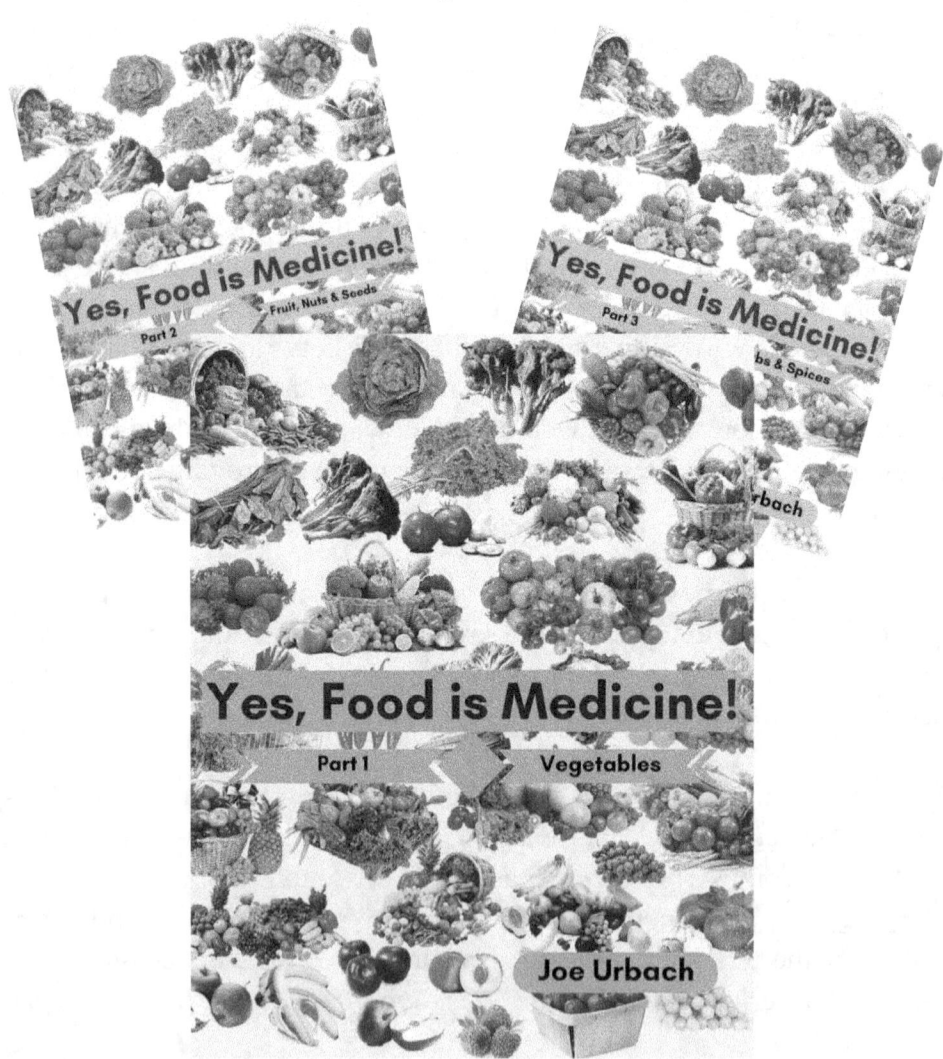

7. Health Benefits of Chocolate

Superfoods don't just come from your supermarket's produce aisle. In fact, those chocolate candy bars next to the gummy bears may now qualify. Study after study proves that dark chocolate—sweet, rich, and delicious—is good for more than curing a broken heart. The secret behind its powerful punch is cacao, also the source of the sweet's distinct taste. Packed with healthy chemicals like flavonoids and theobromine, this little bean is a disease-killing bullet. The only problem? Cacao on its own is bitter, chalky, nasty stuff.

Theobroma Cacao, the Latin name for chocolate, means "Food of the Gods" for a good reason. It's a heavenly way to lift your performance. I am not talking about the "junk" chocolate in candy bars and sweet desserts; No, I am talking about dark chocolate which has a long history of being used as a healing plant, a mood enhancer, and even an aphrodisiac. So, you're in luck: you can indeed use high quality chocolate to take delicious control of your own biology!

Chocolate has gotten a lot of media coverage in recent years because it's believed that it may help protect your cardiovascular system. The reasoning is that the cocoa bean is rich in a class of plant nutrients called flavonoids.

- **Flavonoids -** help protect plants from environmental toxins and help repair damage. They can be found in a variety of foods, such as fruits and vegetables. When we eat foods rich in flavonoids, it appears that we also benefit from this "antioxidant" power.
- **Antioxidants -** are believed to help the body's cells resist damage caused by free radicals that are formed by normal bodily processes, such as breathing, and from environmental contaminants, like cigarette smoke. If your body does not have enough antioxidants to combat the amount of oxidation that occurs, it can become damaged by free radicals. For example, an increase in oxidation can cause low-density lipoprotein (LDL), also known as "bad" cholesterol, to form plaque on the artery walls.
- **Flavanols -** are the main type of flavonoid found in cocoa and chocolate. In addition to having antioxidant qualities, research shows that flavanols have other potential influences on vascular health, such as lowering blood pressure, improving blood flow to the brain and heart, and making blood platelets less sticky and able to clot.

Now, you may have heard that chocolate affects your brain by causing the release of the "happiness neurotransmitters" – serotonin, dopamine, and endorphins. Like coffee, chocolate is also a potent source of polyphenol antioxidants. But experienced chocolate hackers also know chocolate to be a useful tool for improving performance in lesser-known ways. In fact, cacao exerts a systemic effect on the body, with benefits ranging from improved healthy blood flow and cognition to beneficial alterations in gut bacteria! Here are some of the most important benefits of chocolate (besides taste…).

1. High Pressure Mood Improver?

One of the most alluring effects of chocolate consumption is its improvement in mood. Your mood matters even more when you're stressed. Luckily, chocolate can help even in high-pressure situations, according to one study. Participants were asked to complete serial subtraction tasks of threes and sevens (counting down by 3s and 7s), and a rapid visual information-processing task to test sustained attention. Those who consumed cocoa flavanol drinks prior to the trial had overall better cognitive performance and reported less 'mental fatigue' than the control group.

2. Chocolate makes you eat less?

One of my favorite effects of chocolate consumption is a reduction in appetite. One study quantified this by giving participants a 100g serving of either milk chocolate or dark chocolate two hours before being served an all-you-can-eat lunch. Ingestion of dark chocolate was correlated with a 17% lower calorie intake at the following meal, compared to the milk chocolate group.

3. Maintenance of a Healthy Cardiovascular System

Regular chocolate consumption is also associated with improved markers for cardiovascular health. Notably, the polyphenols in cacao increase HDL cholesterol (the good kind), which in turns leads to decreased oxidized LDL cholesterol (the bad kind). Other effects include higher levels of circulating nitric oxide, and reduced platelet adhesion, resulting in improved endothelial function.

One study even found the particular cacao flavanol epicatechin to be responsible for the rise in nitric oxide, which is essential for vascular health. Bioavailability of nitric oxide is an essential determinate of vascular health as it regulates dilation tone, signals cell growth and inflammatory response, and protects blood vessels from clotting.

Importantly, vascular function profoundly modulates insulin-regulated glucose uptake, thus, it should come as no surprise that dark chocolate consumption also improves healthy levels of insulin sensitivity.

4. Chocolate makes your skin glow…and may reduce sunburn?

Another cool thing chocolate does is help you maintain healthy skin by modulating healthy blood flow. In one study, two groups of women consumed either a high flavanol or low flavanol cocoa powder for a period of 12 weeks. While the low flavanol group showed no change in markers of skin health, subjects in the high flavanol group had on average 25% reduction in UV-induced erythema (sunburn) after exposure to a solar simulator. Additionally, the high flavanol group recorded increased skin density and thickness, as well as better hydration and less transepidermal water loss.

5. Healthy Inflammation Levels from Powerful Antioxidants

Chocolate has inflammation-modulating properties. In one study, obese mice supplemented with cocoa powder had healthier levels of inflammation and insulin. These mice also had a 30% reduction in plasma levels of the major pro-inflammatory mediator interleukin 6.

6. Chocolate is a prebiotic!

While many studies assume that it is the cacao polyphenols acting directly to modulate biomarkers, it is most likely the case that at least some of the effect is indirect, and works through interaction with our gut microbiome. Research suggests that low molecular weight cocoa flavanols such as epicatechin and catechin can be absorbed directly into blood circulation, (unless you mix them with milk) but this is not so for the larger polyphenols. In this case, microflora in the colon work to break down high molecular weight polyphenols, so that the smaller secondary metabolites may circulate throughout the body.

If gut bacteria are feeding on the larger cocoa polyphenols, then it follows that the composition of the intestinal microbiome will be altered. In fact, one study did discover a beneficial prebiotic effect of high flavanol chocolate consumption. After a period of 4 weeks of consuming a high flavanol cocoa powder, subjects had a significant increase in bifidobacterial and lactobacilli populations, as well as significantly decreased clostridia levels. This was accompanied by significantly decreased C-reactive protein (which correlates to inflammation reduction in the body), which was associated particularly with changes in lactobacilli.

7. Cellular Rejuvenation (Anti-Aging)

Last, but certainly not least, cacao can enhance mitochondrial biogenesis, or, the creation of new mitochondria! It is the flavanol epicatechin in chocolate which is responsible for mitogenesis. In one study, oral administration of epicatechin to senile mice shifted numerous biomarkers towards those of young mice, including sirtuin 1, a well-recognized regulator of mitochondrial biogenesis. In another mouse study, treatment with epicatechin improved exercise performance by 50% compared to controls, and enhanced muscle fatigue resistance by 30%.

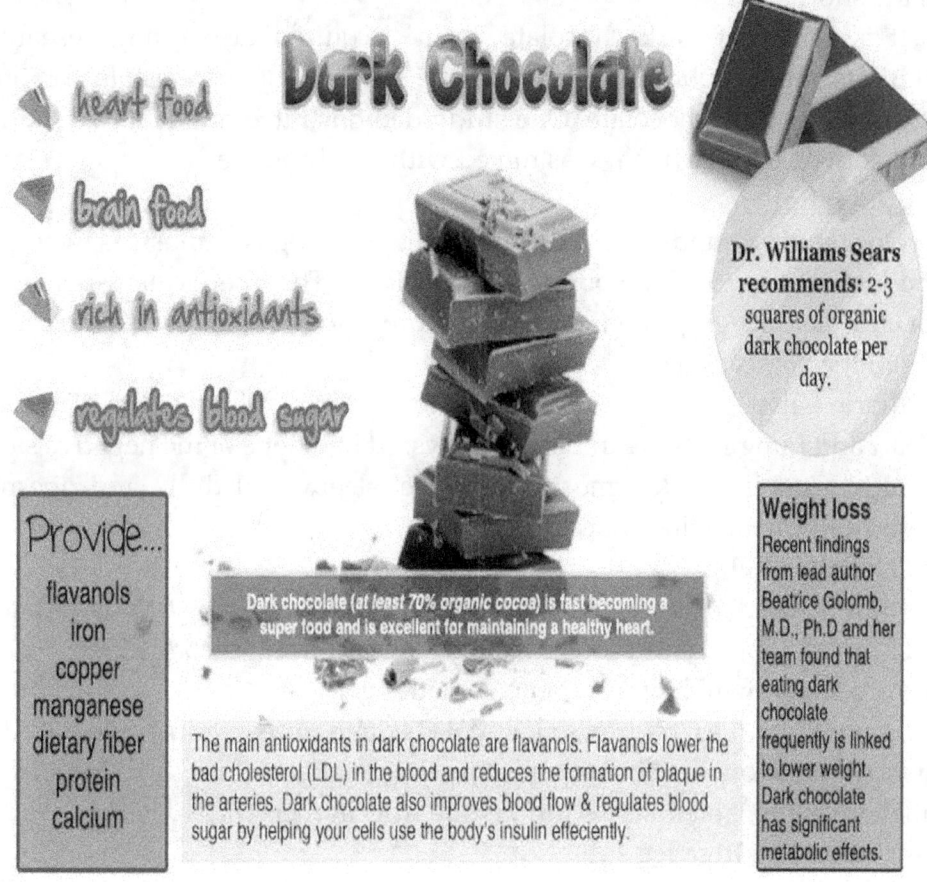

Dark Chocolate

- heart food
- brain food
- rich in antioxidants
- regulates blood sugar

Dr. Williams Sears recommends: 2-3 squares of organic dark chocolate per day.

Provide...
flavanols
iron
copper
manganese
dietary fiber
protein
calcium

Dark chocolate (*at least 70% organic cocoa*) is fast becoming a super food and is excellent for maintaining a healthy heart.

The main antioxidants in dark chocolate are flavanols. Flavanols lower the bad cholesterol (LDL) in the blood and reduces the formation of plaque in the arteries. Dark chocolate also improves blood flow & regulates blood sugar by helping your cells use the body's insulin efficiently.

Weight loss
Recent findings from lead author Beatrice Golomb, M.D., Ph.D and her team found that eating dark chocolate frequently is linked to lower weight. Dark chocolate has significant metabolic effects.

8. Cognitive Improvement

The good news isn't over yet. Dark chocolate may also improve the function of the brain. One study of healthy volunteers showed that 5 days of consuming high-flavanol cocoa improved blood flow to the brain. Cocoa may also significantly improve cognitive function in elderly people with mental impairment. It also improves verbal fluency and several risk factors for disease. Cocoa also contains stimulant substances like caffeine and theobromine, which may be a key reason cocoa can improve brain function in the short term

It is said that dark chocolate is an "acquired taste," and research suggests that theobromine may be the component responsible for our attraction to dark chocolate. One study demonstrated an increased liking for a 'novel' drink when it was mixed with theobromine.

9. Cough Relief

One study found that chocolate quieted coughs almost as well as codeine, thanks to the theobromine it contains. This chemical, responsible for chocolate's feel-good effect, may suppress activity in a part of the brain called the vagus nerve.

Maria Belvisi, a professor of respiratory pharmacology at the National Heart and Lung Institute in London, says, "It had none of the negative side effects." Codeine makes most people feel sleepy and dull—and doesn't taste anything like fine chocolate.

10. Diarrhea Relief

Both South American and European cultures have a history that dates back to the 16th century of treating diarrhea with cocoa. Modern-day science has shown they were onto something.

Scientists at the Children's Hospital Oakland Research Institute found that cocoa flavonoids bind to a protein that regulates fluid secretion in the small intestine, potentially stopping the trots in their tracks.

11. Higher Intelligence

Next time you're under pressure on a work project, don't feel so guilty about grabbing a dark chocolate bar from the vending machine. Not only will it help your body ward off the effects of stress, but it'll boost your brain power when you really need it.

A University of Nottingham researcher found that drinking cocoa rich in flavanols boosts blood flow to key parts of the brain for 2 to 3 hours, which could improve performance and alertness in the short term.

Other researchers from Oxford University and Norway looked at chocolate's long-term effects on the brain by studying the diets of more than 2,000 people over age 70. They found that those who consumed flavanol-rich chocolate, wine, or tea scored significantly higher on cognitive tests than those who didn't.

12. Diabetes Prevention

Candy as a diabetes foe? Sure enough. In a small Italian study, participants who ate a candy bar's worth of dark chocolate once a day for 15 days saw their potential for insulin resistance drop by nearly half. "Flavonoids increase nitric oxide production," says lead researcher Claudio Ferri, M.D., a professor at the University of L'Aquila in Italy. "And that helps control insulin sensitivity."

What about all of the fat in chocolate?

You may be surprised to learn that chocolate isn't as bad for you as once believed. The fat in chocolate comes from cocoa butter and is made up of equal amounts of oleic acid (a heart-healthy monounsaturated fat also found in olive oil), stearic and palmitic acids. Stearic and palmitic acids are forms of saturated fat. You may know that saturated fats are linked to increases in LDL cholesterol and the risk of heart disease.

But, research shows that stearic acid appears to have a neutral effect on cholesterol, neither raising nor lowering it. Although palmitic acid does affect cholesterol levels, it only makes up one-third of the fat calories in chocolate. Still, this does not mean you can eat all the dark chocolate you'd like.

First, be careful about the type of dark chocolate you choose: chewy caramel-marshmallow-nut-covered dark chocolate is by no means a heart-healthy food option. Watch out for those extra

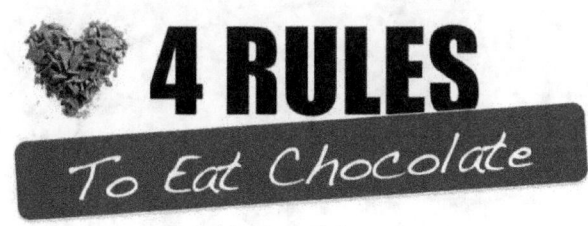

4 RULES To Eat Chocolate

#1 The darker the chocolate, the better.
70% cocoa or more.

#2 Read the ingredients label.
No high-fructose corn syrup
No hydrogenated fat

#3 Avoid milk chocolate products.
Dairy blocks the absorption of antioxidants

#4 Limit the serving size.
15-30g per day

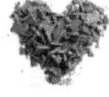

ingredients that can add lots of extra fat and calories. Second, there is currently no established serving size of chocolate to help you reap the cardiovascular benefits it may offer, and more research is needed in this area. However, we do know that you no longer need to feel guilty if you enjoy a small piece of dark chocolate once in a while.

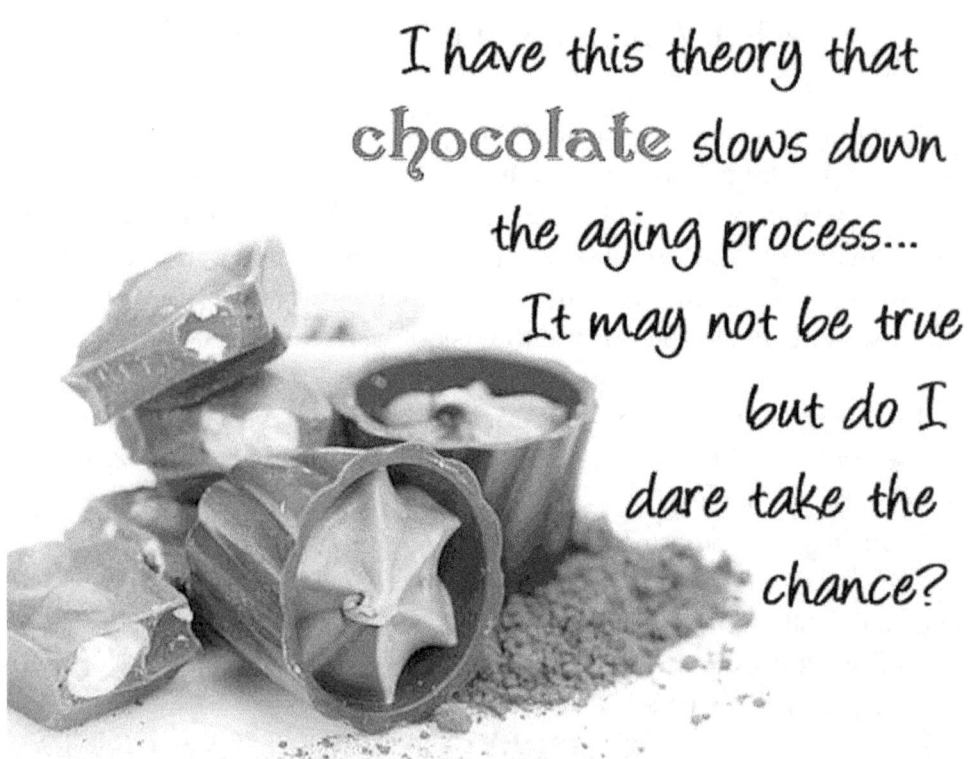

I have this theory that chocolate slows down the aging process... It may not be true but do I dare take the chance?

So, for now, enjoy moderate portions of chocolate (e.g., 1 ounce) a few times per week, and don't forget to eat other flavonoid-rich foods like apples, red wine, tea, onions and cranberries.

8. Health Benefits of Wine

OK, so you pop open the cork after a killer day at work, and the luscious wine flows in mellow drops into your glass. Then this voice whispers in your ear. "Should I be drinking wine?" You try to make healthy food choices and go to the gym and yoga a few times a week. Are you negating your efforts

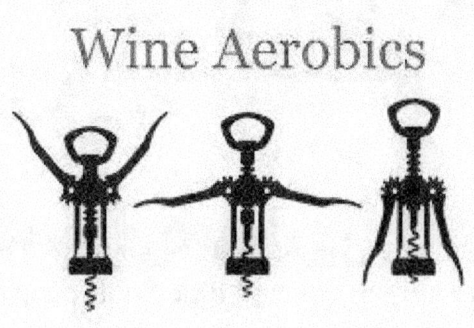

with a few sips? You know that over-indulging is a health no-no, but what about a glass of wine a few times per week?

Unless you've been living under a rock, you've surely heard of the heart-healthy benefits of red wine. Prepare to be amazed. More than just being heart-healthy, wine has a slew of surprising health benefits, many of which stem from resveratrol. Some plants make resveratrol to fight off bacteria and fungi, or to withstand a drought or lack of nutrients. Red and purple grapes, blueberries, cranberries, mulberries, peanuts, and pistachios are sources. Resveratrol may be the *wonder ingredient* responsible for many of wine's benefits. Isolating the resveratrol does not yield the same powers, indicating that a constellation of forces act together to protect the body. Most studies focus on the benefits of red wine because white grapes do not contain resveratrol. (More on resveratrol in just a bit.)

So, as I said above, prepare to be amazed but also prepare to be relieved. You're about to learn how a wine-drinking ritual can be a powerful health elixir. Check out the following benefits of wine that go way beyond heart healthiness.

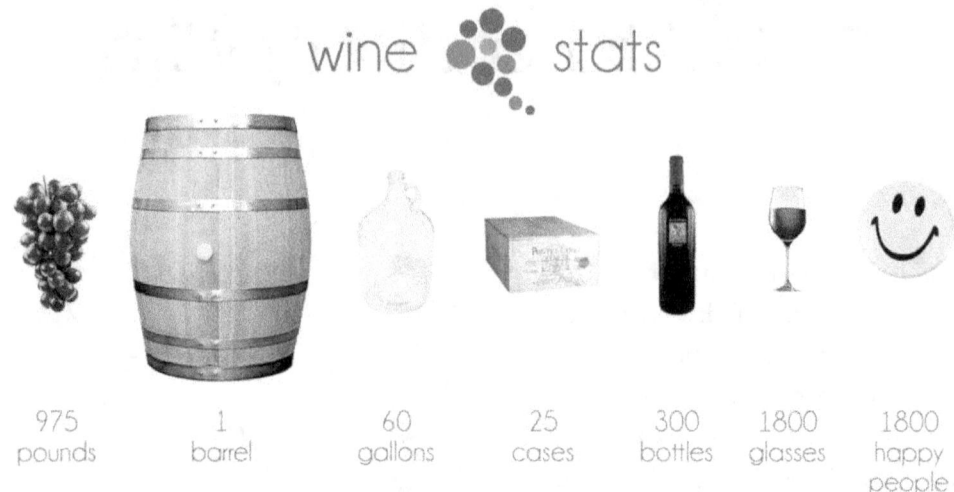

wine stats

975 pounds	1 barrel	60 gallons	25 cases	300 bottles	1800 glasses	1800 happy people

1. So, You just might Live Longer - That's right. On the island of Ikarios, a recently discovered Blue Zone, people live longer than anywhere else in the world. Daily wine consumption is part of a dietary pattern that encourages long life through eating fewer animal-based foods and eating more plant-based foods. You'll find the long-lived residents of Crete and Sardinia sipping dark red wine, a part of their anti-aging lifestyle. A 2007 study suggests procyanidins, compounds found in red wine tannins, help promote cardiovascular health. Wines produced in areas of southwest France and Sardinia, where people tend to live longer, have particularly high concentrations of the compound.

Researchers at Harvard Medical School uncovered evidence that resveratrol directly activates a protein that promotes health and longevity in animal models. Resveratrol increases the activity of sirtuins (longevity pathways), a group of genes that protects the body from diseases of aging.

2. Want to Improve Your Memory – Have some wine, resveratrol may help improve short-term memory. After just 30 minutes of testing, researchers found that participants taking resveratrol had a significant increase in retention of words and showed faster performance in the portion of the brain associated with the formation of new memories, learning, and emotions.

3. Banish Breakouts with Wine - Resveratrol is able to inhibit the growth of acne-causing bacteria longer than benzoyl peroxide. And it works even better when combined with benzoyl peroxide. So far, drinking the antioxidant is the best way to benefit from its properties. Topical application in creams has not been proven as effective – so imbibe your antioxidants in wine, fruits, and veggies rather than buying expensive creams. Fight pimples and blemishes from the inside out!

4. Wine Better Than a Trip to the Gym - Would you rather drink wine or slave away at the gym? Scientists at the University of Alberta in Canada found that resveratrol improves heart, brain, and bone function; the same way these parts are improved when you go to the gym. Now imagine the benefits of doing both! You see what I did there right? I am not advocating you stop exercising, I just want you to add a little wine to your routine!

5. Banish the Blues - You know wine helps you relax… but what about depression? Researchers in Spain have found that men and women who drank two to seven glasses of wine per week, were less likely to be diagnosed with depression. Even when taking into account lifestyle factors which could influence their findings, the reduced risk held strong.

6. Reduce (not increase) Risk of Liver Disease - This study challenged conventional thinking about alcohol and liver disease. Modest wine consumption, defined as one glass per day, may decrease the prevalence of Non-Alcoholic Fatty Liver Disease (NAFLD). Modest wine drinkers, as compared to tee-totalers, cut their risk of NAFLD in half.

7. Healthy Eyes - Resveratrol stops out-of-control blood vessel growth in the eyes, according to Washington University School of Medicine in St. Louis. This may help with treatment of diabetic retinopathy and age-related macular degeneration. Note that these studies were done in mice, so the dose for humans is not yet clear. But this is a great start.

8. Protect your pearly whites

8. Wine Protects You're Pearly Whites - Did you know that drinking wine is a little-known way to protect your teeth from bacteria? I mentioned wine's antimicrobial effects on the skin. Well, it also helps reduce bacteria on our teeth. Using five of the common oral plaque-causing bacteria, scientists noted almost complete degradation of the bacteria after applying the biofilms with red wine.

9. Cut Multiple Cancer Risks –

- **Breast Cancer:** Red grapes are the fruit best able to suppress the activity of aromatase, the enzyme used by breast tumors to produce their own estrogen – this is called an aromatase inhibitor. Red wine may serve as a nutritional aromatase inhibitor, which may ameliorate the elevated breast cancer risk associated with alcohol intake. Note that you can also eat red grapes; those with seeds are especially helpful. Resveratrol is also thought to kill cancer cells by cutting off a pathway that feeds cancer cells.
- **Colon Cancer:** Studies show that moderate consumption of red wine can reduce the risk of colon cancer by 50%.
- **Prostate Cancer:** Harvard Men's Health Watch reports that men who drink an average of four to seven glasses of red wine per week have a 52% less chance of being diagnosed with prostate cancer compared to those who don't drink wine.

Red wine appears particularly protective against advanced or aggressive cancers. Doctors speculate that flavonoids and resveratrol contain potent antioxidants and may counterbalance androgens, the male hormones that stimulate the prostate.

10. Get Rid of the Sniffles - So maybe grandma's cold remedy isn't so strange after all. A study looked at 4,000 faculty members at five universities across Spain. Those who drank wine were less likely to come down with a cold compared to those that drank beer or spirits. Researchers think that the antioxidants help lower inflammation and reduce the symptoms of colds.

11. Lower Your Cholesterol (without changing your diet) - Resveratrol is thought to reduce LDL and increase HDL, meaning that our blood vessels are less likely to be coated with plaque. Even the American Heart Association admits that moderate consumption of any type of alcohol can increase your HDL, or good cholesterol, by about 12%.

12. Reduce Stroke Risk - Wine may reduce your risk of ischemic stroke. In analyses adjusted for age, sex, and smoking, intake of wine on a monthly, weekly, or daily basis was associated with a lower risk of stroke compared with no wine intake at all.

13. Manage Diabetes with Wine - The polyphenols in red wine interact with cells involved in the development and storage of fat and the regulation of blood sugar. The numbers of polyphenols in a glass of red wine rivals the blood sugar regulating activity of certain diabetes drugs.

14. Slash you Risk of Diabetes - Those who drink moderately have a 30% lower risk of Type 2 diabetes. This may be due to the polyphenols mentioned above or again to resveratrol, which improves sensitivity to insulin. Insulin resistance is the most important critical factor contributing to Type 2 diabetes risk.

The monumental mistake people make is trying to buy these benefits in a pill, rather than looking at how wine can be a part of a healthy lifestyle. We want to bottle it, sell it, and find that magic bullet. **Supplements have not proven to have the benefits of simple foods**. Nature is complex, and we haven't figured out how to put that in a pill (and I hope we don't). The most important thing you can do is start to look at the big picture. Think of the slow-paced life of the Mediterranean and bring a little bit of that into your life. Take time to prepare a simple meal packed with delicious fresh vegetables and smaller portions of red meat. Savor this meal. Linger at the table with your friends and family. And of course – enjoy a leisurely glass of wine without feeling guilty!

Resveratrol, Resveratrol, Resveratrol. What is it?

Resveratrol is a compound found in some plants. Plants produce resveratrol to fight off bacteria and fungi. Resveratrol also protects plants from ultraviolet irradiation. Red wine contains more resveratrol than white wine because it is fermented with the skins (white wine is not). Most of the resveratrol in grapes is in the seeds and skin.

The following plants and drinks are rich in resveratrol

- Red wine
- Grapes
- Blueberries
- Raspberries
- Bilberries
- Peanuts

The health benefits linked to moderate wine consumption are mostly due to the beverage's resveratrol content.

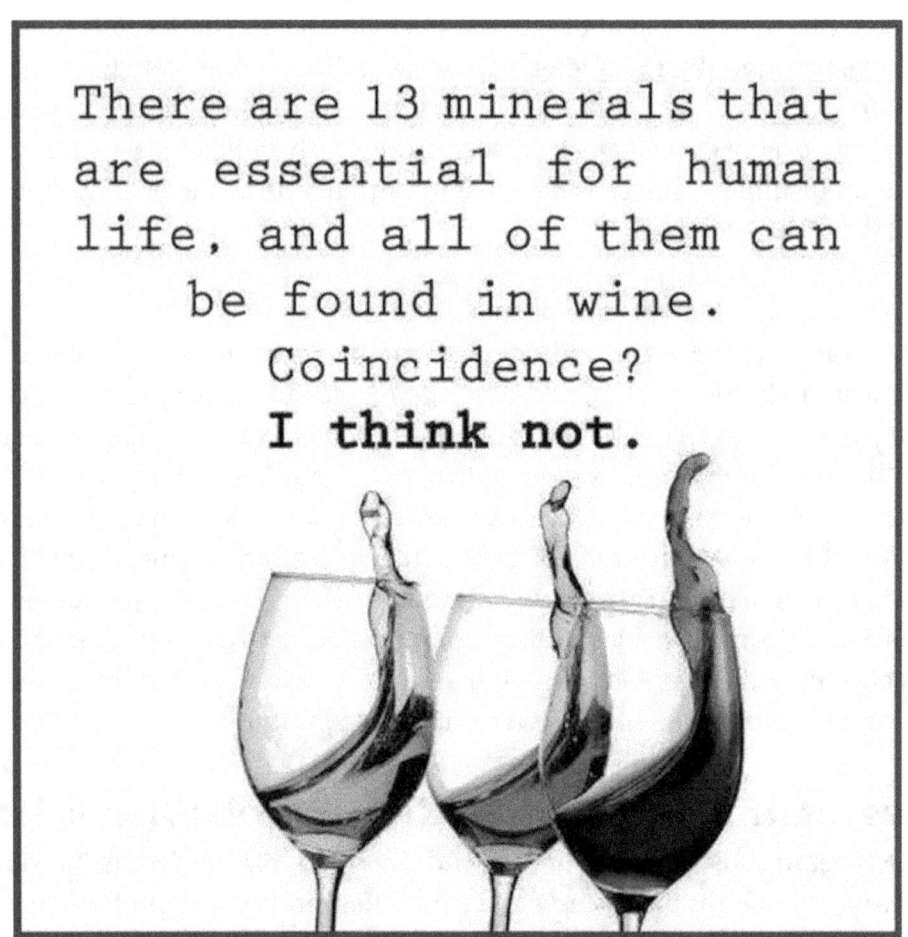

There are 13 minerals that are essential for human life, and all of them can be found in wine. Coincidence? **I think not.**

Wine, especially the red variety, has been studied extensively over many years with impressive findings suggesting it may promote a longer lifespan, protect against certain cancers, improve mental health, provide benefits to the heart, and offers many other health benefits as well.

9. Chocolate & Alcoholism

While researching this book, I learned that recovering alcoholics, especially those who are early in the recovery process, are encouraged to eat chocolate to curb their craving for alcohol. According to my research, this recommendation is included in the book, *Alcoholics Anonymous*, which is also known as "The Big Book" to those who are in recovery. Why is this?

Some people hypothesize that chocolate is helpful because it contains a variety of alkaloids that are linked to alcoholism, so by eating chocolate, the alcoholic can get these same substances without ingesting alcohol. Further, it is hypothesized that these same biochemicals cause "chocolate addiction." But in investigating this claim regarding "chocolate addiction" further, it came to my attention that this phenomenon is nothing more than wishful thinking. In fact, a researcher presented this very argument at an upcoming meeting in England.

Of course, this scientist is making an argument based on other people's research, but his argument is based upon the fact that, even though chocolate contains pharmacologically significant amounts of theobromine, phenylethylamine, tryptophan and anandamide, there are plenty of other foods out there that contain these same substances, and in greater quantities than does chocolate, yet these other foods are not considered nearly as "addictive" as chocolate.

But to understand this argument more fully, it is first important to understand what these biochemicals do when they are in your body. Theobromine is structurally related to caffeine, but is a much less powerful stimulant than what you get in a cup of coffee. Additionally, due to dilution, theobromine concentrations are very, very low in chocolate and thus, are not physiologically significant.

Phenylethylamine is another stimulant found in chocolate. Its molecular structure is similar to amphetamine, and it also induces an elevated mood. However, it is not known how much (if any) of this substance actually reaches the brain after passing through the powerful acid-bath in the stomach.

Another biochemical, tryptophan, is actually an essential amino acid, which is involved in the production of serotonin. Serotonin is a neurotransmitter that causes people to feel calm and satisfied. However, there are plenty of other food sources that also provide tryptophan in pharmacologically significant concentrations, but they aren't foods that people typically associate with "addition".

Anandamide acts similarly to marijuana to produce an emotional "high" by binding to the THC receptor in the brain. However, like phenylethylamine, stomach acids probably destroy it before it manages to reach one's brain THC receptors to trigger any happiness.

So, based on this information, Peter Rogers of the University of Bristol in England argues at the annual BA Festival of Science, held at the University of York, that because these other foods are not addictive, chocolate likewise is not addictive. (However, let me point out that Rogers is not the first person to make this argument).

"A more compelling explanation lies in our ambivalent attitudes towards chocolate," Rogers said. "It is highly desired but should be eaten with restraint (nice but naughty). Our unfulfilled desire to eat chocolate, resulting from restraint, is thus experienced as craving, which in turn is attributed to 'addiction.'"

Currently, milk chocolate is the world's best-selling variety of chocolate, for reasons that escape me: some people, like me, prefer our chocolate to be *dark*.

But in his presenation, Rogers instead argued that chocolate's appeal is due to the sugar and fat it contains. Unfortunately, one argument that Rogers apparently will not address is how chocolate and the substances it contains are capable of relieving one's craving for alcohol.

Conclusion
In my humble opinion

Look, while I could bow to convention and follow the "rules" of proper book layout and publishing, those that demand that in the conclusion I sum up all of the preceding chapters and answer any questions that may still remain in the minds of my readers, I would rather not.

Frankly I just don't want to do that. So, since I have never much been one for following all the "rules," I think I'll just approach this conclusion the way I want.

You see, I absolutely do not want to answer all of your questions with this book. In fact, I think that all of those so called, "all you need to know" books are ridiculous!

What I want to achieve with this work, what hope I have achieved is that I provided you with enough solid, scientific information that you are encouraged to start asking more questions about chocolate, wine, and beer; their history, their impact on mankind, and their possible impact on your health. I hope you do some additional research of your own!

As for how I would sum up this book? Let me simply paraphrase something I said many times earlier in this work…

Too much of a good thing is not a good thing! Increased alcohol consumption over time will not lead to better health but could, in fact, ruin your health. What's more the same is true for the unchecked consumption of chocolate!

Moderation is the key word here!

I will leave you with just a few more bits of graphical information to consider:

This is what one drink looks like

According to the Dietary Guidelines for Americans, moderate drinking is up to one drink per day for women and up to two drinks per day for men. A standard drink contains 14 grams of pure alcohol.

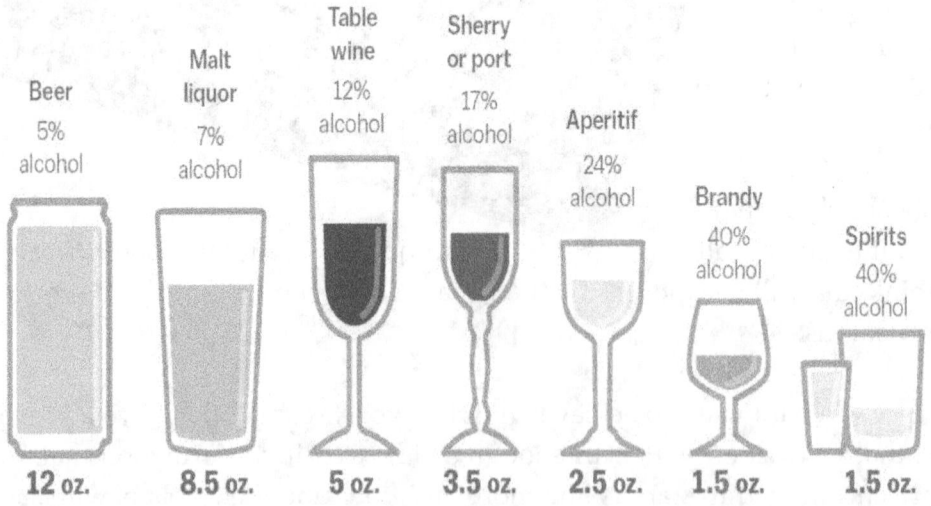

Measures are approximate, since different brands and beverages may vary in their actual alcohol content.

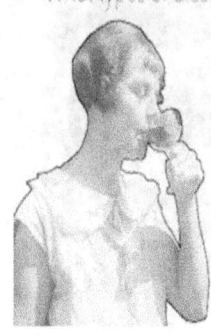

What types of alcohol do U.S. adults prefer?

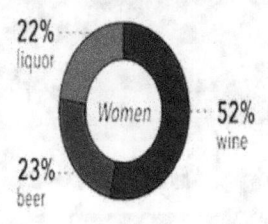

22%
liquor

Women

52%
wine

23%
beer

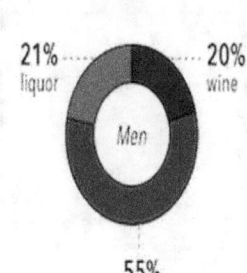

21%
liquor

20%
wine

Men

55%
beer

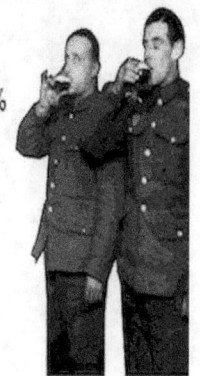

STANDARD-SIZED DRINK EQUIVALENTS
APPROXIMATE NUMBER OF STANDARD-SIZED DRINKS IN:

BEER or COOLER

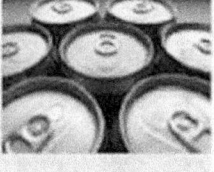

12 oz.
~5% alcohol

- 12 oz. = 1
- 16 oz. = 1.3
- 22 oz. = 2
- 40 oz. = 3.3

TABLE WINE

5 oz.
~12% alcohol

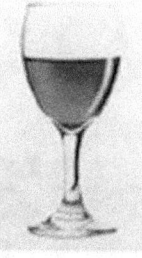

- a 750 mL (25 oz.) bottle = 5

MALT LIQUOR

8–9 oz.
~7% alcohol

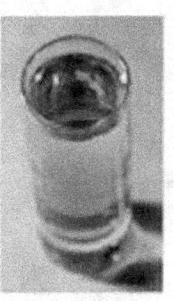

- 12 oz. = 1.5
- 16 oz. = 2
- 22 oz. = 2.5
- 40 oz. = 4.5

80-proof SPIRITS
(hard liquor)

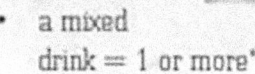

1.5 oz.
~40% alcohol

- a mixed drink = 1 or more*
- a pint (16 oz.) = 11
- a fifth (25 oz.) = 17
- 1.75 L (59 oz.) = 39

123

Most popular varieties of table wine in the U.S. by market share

Chardonnay *21%*

Cabernet Sauvignon *12%*

Merlot *9%*

Pinot Grigio/Gris *8%*

WINE SALES IN THE U.S.

Year	Millions of 9-liter cases of wine	Total retail value
2008	313.8	$30 billion
2009	321.1	$28.7 billion
2010	329.7	$30 billion
2011	351.5	$32.9 billion
2012	360.1	$34.6 billion

WHICH IS HEALTHIER?

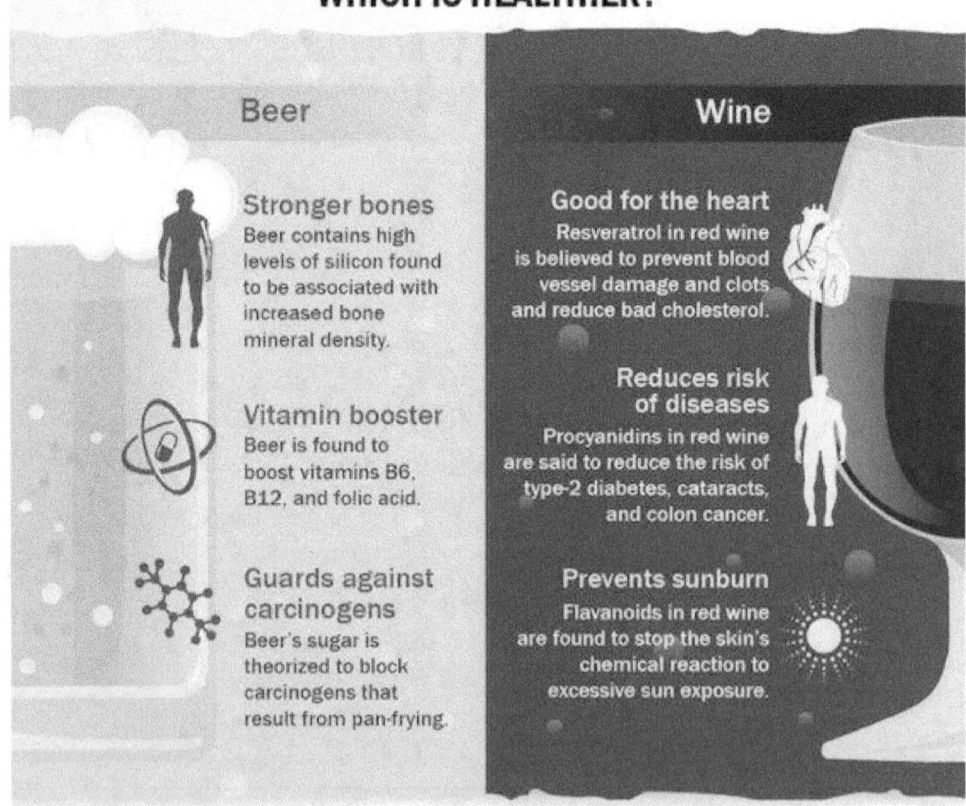

Beer

Stronger bones
Beer contains high levels of silicon found to be associated with increased bone mineral density.

Vitamin booster
Beer is found to boost vitamins B6, B12, and folic acid.

Guards against carcinogens
Beer's sugar is theorized to block carcinogens that result from pan-frying.

Wine

Good for the heart
Resveratrol in red wine is believed to prevent blood vessel damage and clots and reduce bad cholesterol.

Reduces risk of diseases
Procyanidins in red wine are said to reduce the risk of type-2 diabetes, cataracts, and colon cancer.

Prevents sunburn
Flavanoids in red wine are found to stop the skin's chemical reaction to excessive sun exposure.

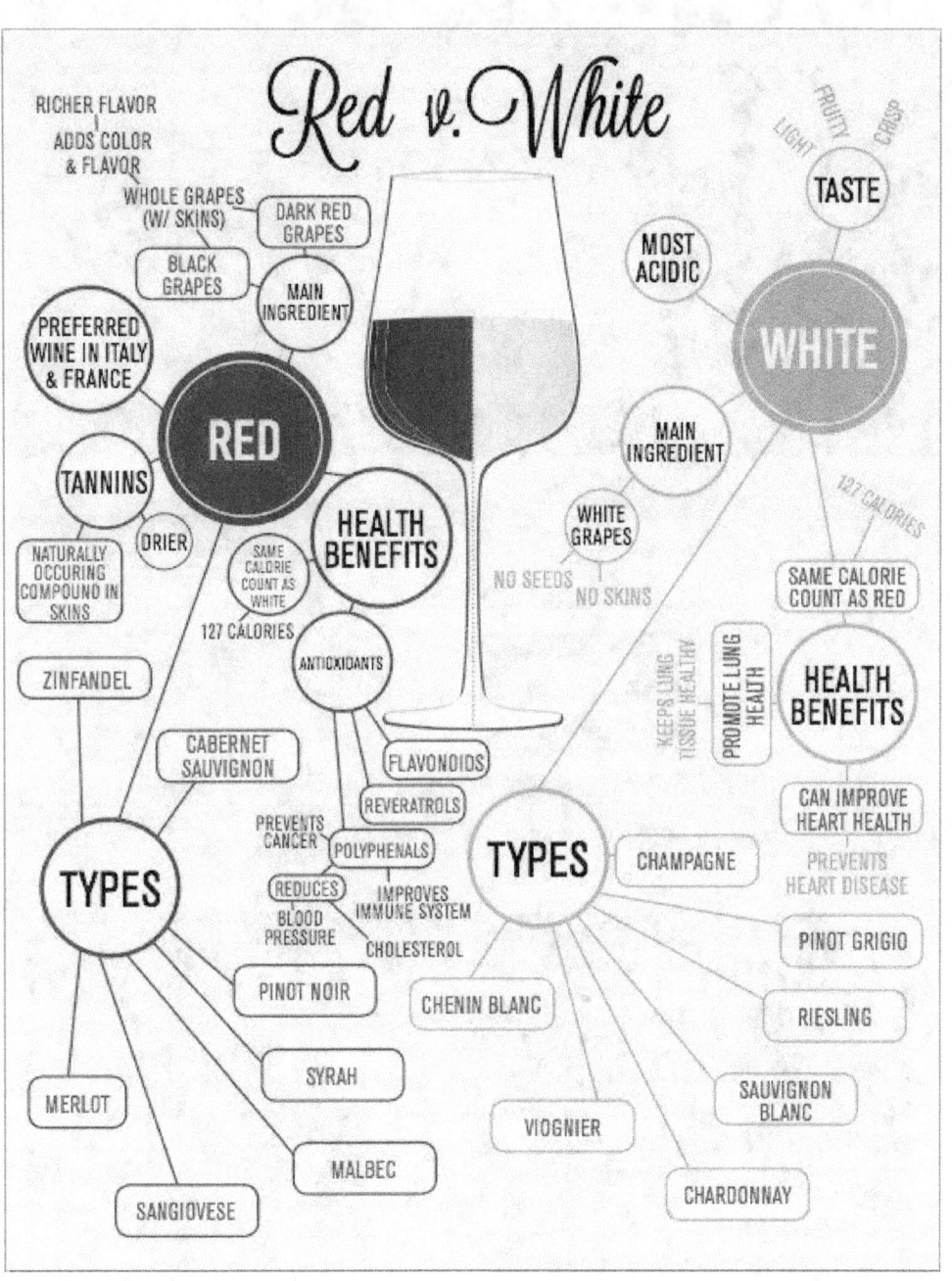

Red v. White

RED

- RICHER FLAVOR
- ADDS COLOR & FLAVOR
- WHOLE GRAPES (W/ SKINS)
- DARK RED GRAPES
- BLACK GRAPES
- MAIN INGREDIENT
- PREFERRED WINE IN ITALY & FRANCE
- TANNINS
  - DRIER
  - NATURALLY OCCURING COMPOUND IN SKINS

HEALTH BENEFITS
- SAME CALORIE COUNT AS WHITE
- 127 CALORIES
- ANTIOXIDANTS
  - FLAVONOIDS
  - REVERATROLS
  - POLYPHENALS
    - PREVENTS CANCER
    - REDUCES BLOOD PRESSURE
    - IMPROVES IMMUNE SYSTEM
    - CHOLESTEROL

TYPES
- ZINFANDEL
- CABERNET SAUVIGNON
- PINOT NOIR
- MERLOT
- SYRAH
- MALBEC
- SANGIOVESE

WHITE

- LIGHT
- FRUITY
- CRISP
- TASTE
- MOST ACIDIC
- MAIN INGREDIENT
  - WHITE GRAPES
  - NO SEEDS
  - NO SKINS
- 127 CALORIES
- SAME CALORIE COUNT AS RED
- KEEPS LUNG TISSUE HEALTHY
- PROMOTE LUNG HEALTH

HEALTH BENEFITS
- CAN IMPROVE HEART HEALTH
- PREVENTS HEART DISEASE

TYPES
- CHAMPAGNE
- PINOT GRIGIO
- RIESLING
- SAUVIGNON BLANC
- CHARDONNAY
- VIOGNIER
- CHENIN BLANC

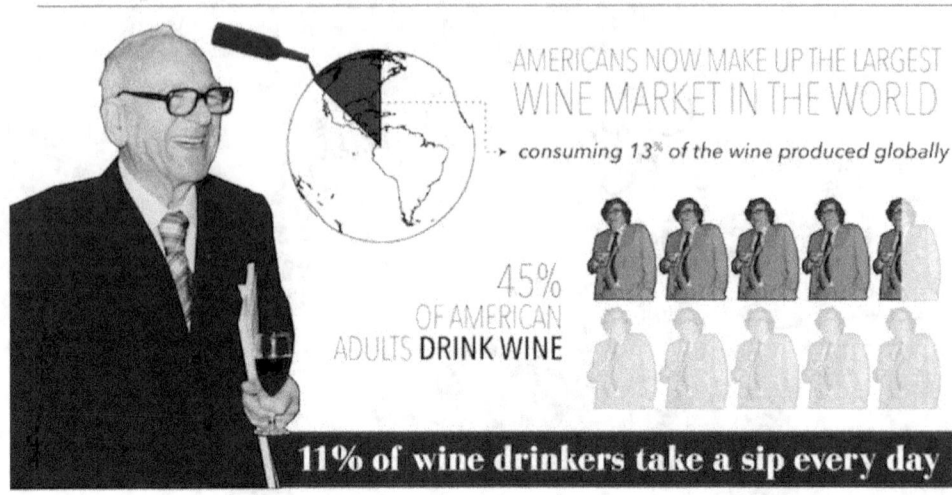

AMERICANS NOW MAKE UP THE LARGEST
WINE MARKET IN THE WORLD

→ *consuming 13% of the wine produced globally*

45%
OF AMERICAN
ADULTS **DRINK WINE**

11% of wine drinkers take a sip every day

WINE CONSUMPTION IN THE U.S.

Year	Wine per resident	Total gallons
2008	2.45 gals	746 million
2009	2.49 gals	763 million
2010	2.53 gals	784 million
2011	2.68 gals	836 million
2012	2.73 gals	856 million

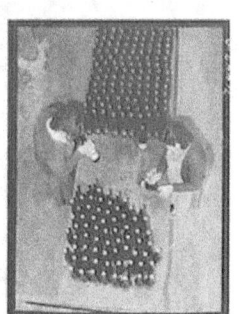

DRINKERS vs NON-DRINKERS

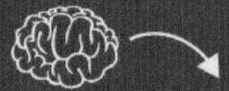

BRAIN function declines at a markedly faster rate in nondrinkers than in moderate drinkers.

MODERATE DRINKERS ARE:

50% less likely to have strokes.

30% less likely to develop type 2 diabetes.

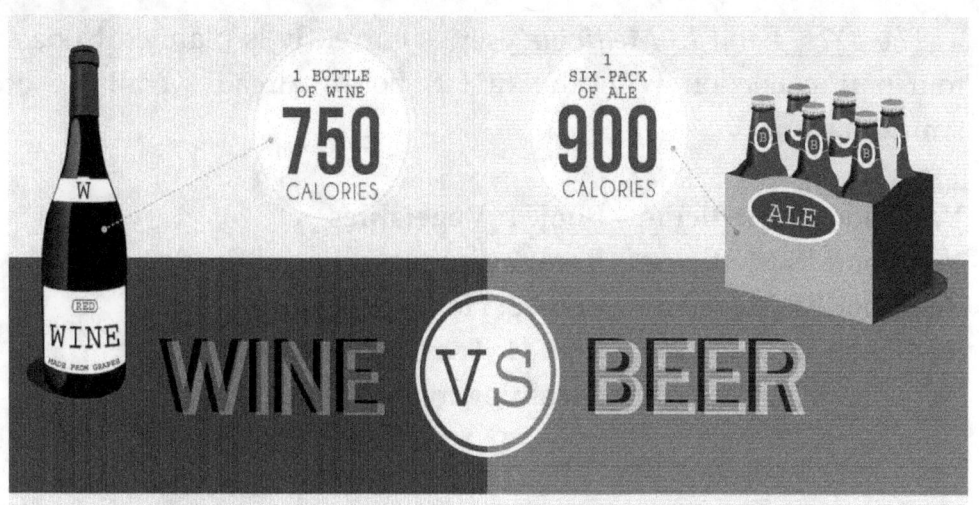

1 BOTTLE OF WINE
750 CALORIES

1 SIX-PACK OF ALE
900 CALORIES

WINE (VS) BEER

A CLOSER LOOK AT HEALTH BENEFITS OF BEER & WINE

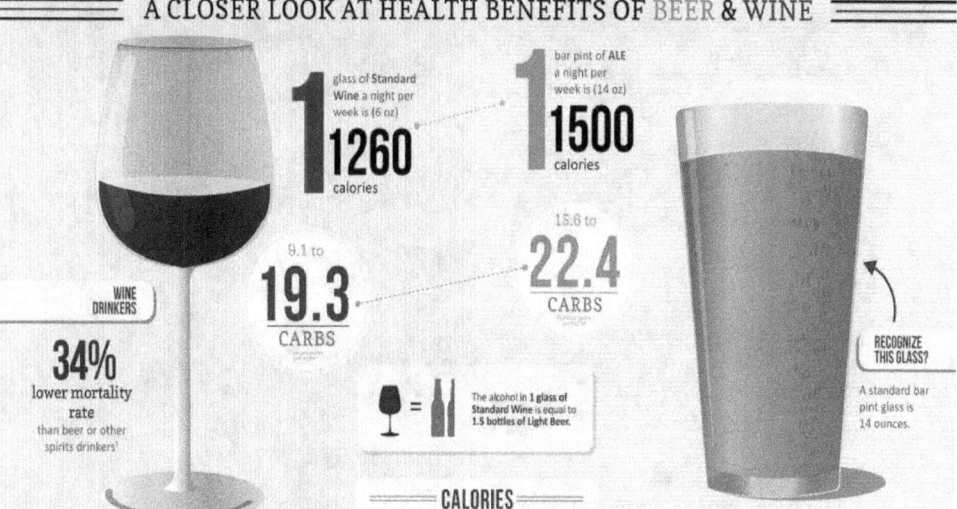

1 glass of Standard Wine a night per week is (6 oz)
1260 calories

1 bar pint of ALE a night per week is (14 oz)
1500 calories

9.1 to
19.3 CARBS

15.6 to
22.4 CARBS

WINE DRINKERS

34% lower mortality rate than beer or other spirits drinkers¹

The alcohol in **1 glass of Standard Wine** is equal to **1.5 bottles of Light Beer.**

RECOGNIZE THIS GLASS?
A standard bar pint glass is 14 ounces.

CALORIES
Wine vs. Beer

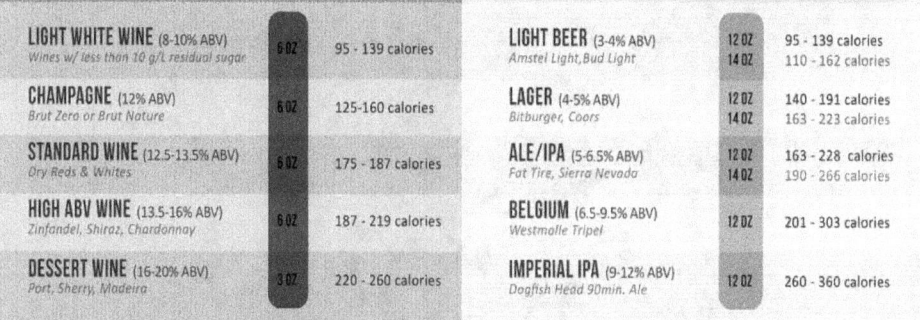

LIGHT WHITE WINE (8-10% ABV) Wines w/ less than 10 g/L residual sugar	6 OZ	95 - 139 calories		**LIGHT BEER** (3-4% ABV) Amstel Light, Bud Light	12 OZ / 14 OZ	95 - 139 calories / 110 - 162 calories
CHAMPAGNE (12% ABV) Brut Zero or Brut Nature	6 OZ	125-160 calories		**LAGER** (4-5% ABV) Bitburger, Coors	12 OZ / 14 OZ	140 - 191 calories / 163 - 223 calories
STANDARD WINE (12.5-13.5% ABV) Dry Reds & Whites	6 OZ	175 - 187 calories		**ALE/IPA** (5-6.5% ABV) Fat Tire, Sierra Nevada	12 OZ / 14 OZ	163 - 228 calories / 190 - 266 calories
HIGH ABV WINE (13.5-16% ABV) Zinfandel, Shiraz, Chardonnay	6 OZ	187 - 219 calories		**BELGIUM** (6.5-9.5% ABV) Westmalle Tripel	12 OZ	201 - 303 calories
DESSERT WINE (16-20% ABV) Port, Sherry, Madeira	3 OZ	220 - 260 calories		**IMPERIAL IPA** (9-12% ABV) Dogfish Head 90min. Ale	12 OZ	260 - 360 calories

The *"Yes, Food IS Medicine"* series currently is planned to be a four-part collection with the first 3 books already available at **Amazon.com:**

Yes, Food IS Medicine – Book 1: Vegetables
Yes, Food IS Medicine – Book 2: Fruits, Nuts and Seeds
Yes, Food IS Medicine – Book 3: Herbs and Spices
Yes, Food IS Medicine – Book 4: Teas and Wild Edibles
(coming in the fall of 2017)

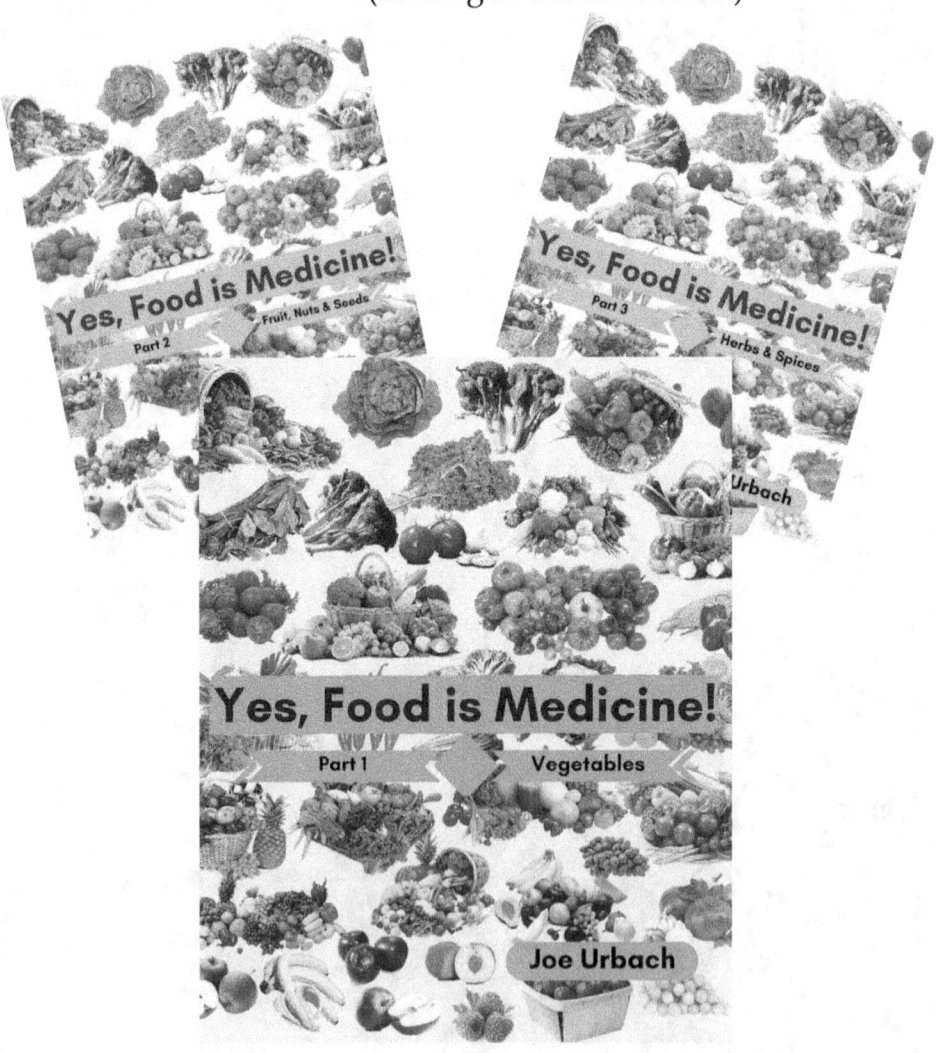